THE MARTIAL WAY AND ITS VIRTUES

We are too late for the gods
and too early for Being.
Being's poem, just begun, is man
                    —*Martin Heidegger*

THE
MARTIAL
WAY AND ITS
VIRTUES
TAO DE GUNG

道德功

F. J. CHU

YMAA Publication Center
Boston, Mass. USA

YMAA Publication Center, Inc.
Main Office
4354 Washington Street
Boston, Massachusetts, 02131
1-800-669-8892 • www.ymaa.com • ymaa@aol.com

10 9 8 7 6 5 4 3 2

Editor: George A. Katchmer Jr.
Illustrations and Chinese Calligraphy: Jerry Fu
Cover Design: Richard Rossiter

Publisher's Cataloging in Publication

Chu, F. J.

The martial way and its virtues : Tao de Gung / F. J. Chu. — 1st ed.
—Boston, Mass. : YMAA Publication Center, 2003

p. ; cm.
Includes bibliographical references and index.
.
ISBN: 1-886969-69-8

1. Martial arts—Moral and ethical aspects. 2. Marial arts—
Psychological aspects. 3. Self-defense— Moral and ethical aspects.
4. Mind and body. I. Title.

GV1102.7.P75 C48 2003   2003109400
796.8/01/9–dc22   0309

Printed in Canada

For
Sifu Carmen Vigliotti, a true warrior
and
Sifu Shue Yiu Kwan, a humble master

CONTENTS

Foreword

My first real insight into the martial arts came somewhat late in life—as a Police Captain in New York City, commanding a precinct in a high crime area. Like many of my contemporaries, my understanding of the martial arts had been limited primarily to my exposure to the antics of the action-movie stars of the 1970's and 80's—Chuck Norris, Bruce Lee, Stephen Seagal, and the like.

Shortly before my assignment to the precinct, its Youth Officer had begun a martial arts program for a group of children in what was arguably the toughest part of the precinct. By the time I moved on to my next assignment, I had seen the program blossom to a point where more than one hundred children were enrolled, coming from several different schools, and interest in the program was still growing.

At the time, precinct commanders were routinely called to headquarters for Crime Control Strategy (or "CompStat") meetings, where we were interrogated about crime conditions in our commands and our plans to address them. At one meeting, as I was describing the martial arts program, the Deputy Commissioner who ran the meetings, an overbearing, albeit effective inquisitor, interrupted me. He smirked, and asked, "You have an increase in assaults—but you're teaching these kids how to fight"?

"No, Commissioner," I replied, "just the opposite. If you came to one of their exhibitions, and saw the discipline, control, confidence, and dedication these children have developed, you would be amazed. That's what the program is about—bringing self-discipline and confidence into these kids' lives."

Indeed it was. These were the children of poverty, growing up in an area where violence was commonplace, the sound of gunshots was routine, and crack vials could be found in almost every doorway. Yet to watch them perform in the exhibitions we held several times a year—to see them move together as a team, listening intently to every command of their instructor; to see the discipline of their individual techniques; to see the intensity and focus of their kicks; to watch the confidence that was beginning to bloom within their souls—sparked hope that they would rise above their surroundings, resist the lure of the many temptations around them, and go on to productive, meaningful lives. That a police officer could be the vessel to inspire such hope was especially impressive, since in this peculiar role he was both samurai and sensei—

the warrior, dedicated to a life of protecting his students and all around them, and the master, passing along precious life lessons to his charges in the guise of techniques for breaking boards.

The experiences of a lifetime in policing have made me particularly sensitive to two themes that are threaded through the pages of this book. The first is that there is, in fact, a perpetual struggle between forces of good and evil in this world—certainly a fact made obvious to everyone who witnessed the devastating attacks of September 11th, 2001, but something known well before that by any police officer who has dealt with death, violence, and the many other manifestations of evil that permeate our society.

The second is that the person best equipped to fight this battle is he or she who has assumed the traits of the warrior described in this book— the intellectual, physical, emotional, and spiritual qualities of The Martial Way. It is he who knows how to fight, and is confident in his abilities, who does not need to. It is he who has accepted and embraced moral principles to guide his life who does not stumble in the face of temptation. It is he who knows and accepts the need of the body and mind for a balance between labor and recreation who can work harder and more productively. It is he who has taken the long, arduous path of integrating all of the many needs of body, mind, and spirit who will quietly lead the way.

I have seen many displays of the calm courage that comes from this discipline of mind and spirit. Perhaps the most striking have been a handful of instances in which I have seen police officers, fired upon or menaced by an adversary, resist the reflexive action of shooting back and effect an arrest without firing a shot, often out of a concern that a stray bullet might strike an innocent bystander. It is hard to find a better example of pure courage, confidence, and the calm that comes from knowing that one is on the side of right and good.

More subtle, perhaps, but of great impact, are the lessons to be learned from those who we call "leaders." The term "leadership" is so broad and ethereal that it almost defies definition—yet there are few concepts that so impact our lives at so many levels, since we are all in some way leaders and followers.

Several years ago, I attended an extensive training seminar on leadership and management conducted by one of the nation's most prestigious business schools. The curriculum drew upon various disciplines in attempting to identify the component parts of the prototype leader.

As I studied the paradigms of leadership that were presented to me via the legends of great leaders of business, the military, government, and labor, I found that the most valuable lesson was to be learned from analyzing the great leaders with whom I have had the good fortune to work—who have been, at various times, my supervisors, my colleagues, and my mentors. I have seen a common pattern of traits in the best of them.

They have all been moral, living their dedication to a set of ethical principals. They have all been compassionate, knowing that life without compassion is empty. They have demanded a high degree of performance, since it is meaningless to strive for anything less than excellence. They have been intelligent and insightful, with knowledge, analytical skills, and judgment continually tested and honed. All have loved laughter, knowing that without humor and enjoyment of life, the rest of one's skills wither.

Two distinct traits come from the same underlying source. They have been fearless—and they have been decisive. Underlying both of these qualities has been extraordinary confidence—the confidence that comes from knowing that one's skills are developed to the highest possible degree, constantly challenged, and based on a moral foundation. They know that they will make mistakes, but that those mistakes will be "of the head" rather than "of the heart." They know that their subordinates or followers will also make mistakes, but they will not rush to either avoid or place blame, because they know that their followers adhere to the same principles and have done their level best to accomplish whatever mission they have been given.

These leaders came from various backgrounds; not all, by any means, have been students of the martial arts. Yet the end result has been the same, by whatever means it was achieved: self-discipline, training, synthesis of the qualities of mind and body in the delicate harmony needed to maximize one's potential.

The mystery is how to develop those qualities in oneself, to rise above the unchallenged, untested, and uninspired. Using the martial arts as its core, *The Martial Way and its Virtues—Tao De Gung*, provides both an insight into the martial arts and a blueprint for a way to begin the journey of achieving mastery of one's body, mind, and spirit. It is a long, arduous, indeed endless journey—but one well worth taking, a journey that will benefit not only the warrior, but also the world.

William R. Connors
Police Commissioner
Rye City, NY

PART I

Prelude

Tao De Gung is a purist's vision of the martial arts. The book is a call to practicing martial artists everywhere and to aspirants of the martial Way. It draws upon the wisdom of the sages, from antiquity to the modern day, to embrace a path of living and training that might be radically different from what one may be pursuing today. The impetus of this essay is the integration of apparently discordant values: pacifism and aggression, mind and body, self-defense and sport, and strategy versus technique. The tension between the meeting of spirituality and brute physical force, and life against death, are recurring themes. *Tao De Gung* highlights the immediate relevance of philosophical thinking on "real life" martial arts practice. Philosophical discourse, like martial arts practice, is a way of life. One becomes a preparatory exercise for the other. Going beyond mere contemplative reflection, it advocates the principle that personal transformation occurs only when it is driven by personal values. These values are then incorporated into a martial artist's life through disciplined and regular practice. Thought embodies action. At the same time, this book seeks to puncture the "illusion of technique" engendered by the many volumes of how-to-fight picture books common in the genre today.

During the long course of training, students of the martial arts occasionally encounter other veteran martial artists who are highly skilled in the art of fighting and self-defense. These individuals are typically the teachers in the training hall and senior instructors at other schools. We admire their technical abilities and seek to learn from their expertise, although we may not necessarily put much stock in their actions outside the martial arts arena. In short, we respect them as fighters even if they may not inspire us as human beings that we model ourselves after.

Alternatively, there are observers and writers of the martial arts scene who bring to bear upon the art an insightful understanding of the historical, philosophical or spiritual underpinnings of the martial Way. On rare occasions we might encounter a few such individuals who, by weight of their wisdom, skill and example, earn our respect as extraordinary human beings. They make a contribution to the understanding and appreciation of the martial arts but may not be competent martial artists themselves. Consequently, their lack of physical and technical proficiency in the martial arts makes us question the real-life applicability and immediacy of what they write or say.

It is uncommon to meet a true martial arts master, and rare to meet a martial arts master who is also a sage. To encounter someone who is arguably qualified to be both is to be in rarefied company. When a martial arts student has the privilege of working with such a person, it is a blessing twice received. In the Chinese worldview, the concept of life-enhancing energy (*chi*) is the foundation of physical conditioning as well as the key to mental empowerment and personal performance. At the highest skill levels, martial arts and spirituality merge. Stated alternatively, at the highest levels the integration of strategy and technique brings about the emergence of spirit and the development of *chi*. Martial arts skill is based on both physical prowess and mental refinement, with an exacting focus on the physical, mental and spiritual being. Thus this book addresses martial artists in training and seekers of the martial Way who choose to make the long, arduous and rewarding journey towards self-perfection, for the martial Way has many invaluable lessons to teach us.

Schopenhauer, one of the most original minds in the history of Western metaphysics, once said: "Live first, then philosophize." What he meant, I believe, is that in order to finally cross over into the realm of true philosophizing, one first must bear all the burdens, learn from all the mistakes, and accept all the frustrations, disappointments and joys of life's long journey.

In that spirit, this book is organized into three parts. Part I sets forth the philosophical precepts of the martial Way as a heroic and enlightened pursuit, one that requires devoted training and ongoing refinement. It puts the martial arts into historical perspective by examining the evolution of one particular martial arts style as it developed from traditional China, to feudal Japan and up through the modern day American scene.

Part II focuses on various aspects of strategy and technique, dwelling upon solitary training and training with partners. These discussions attempt to balance the detailed psychophysical considerations of a violent confrontation with its attendant emotional and attitudinal issues. Topics such as how we should practice, what are the classic mistakes to avoid, how we view ourselves and our opponents, and how we develop our own personalized strategies and techniques are explored. It hints at the real theme of the martial Way as a triumph, not so much against an opponent, but over oneself.

In Part III, the book concludes by returning to the spiritual antecedents of the martial arts. It poses the questions: What are the virtues of martial arts training? What is the philosophical purpose of pursuing the martial Way? This section discusses the development of a warrior mentality and the transformation of a martial artist from student to teacher. It proposes not only how to fight and win—at the risk of enduring damage and loss—but how to win without a fight. To uphold a principle without the physical and moral courage to implement it often renders the practice of a martial code of conduct academic. Finally, the book speculates upon the ideal of an "ultimate convergence" of mind, body and spirit in one person at one given point in time, perhaps generating more questions as well as answers about what kind of martial artist—what kind of person—one wants to become.

One who is good at being a warrior
does not make a show of his might;
One who is good in battle does not get angry;
One who is good at defeating the enemy does not
engage him.

—Lao Tzu

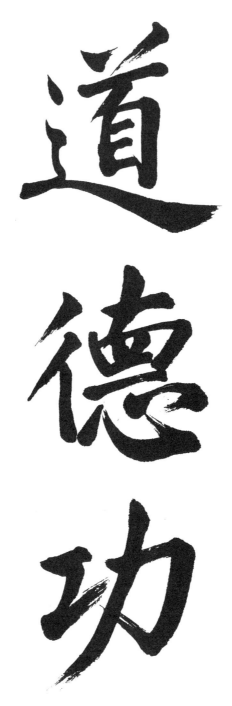

Tao de gung
The martial way and its virtues

The Force of Virtue | I

The wisdom and knowledge that the martial arts offer is something that should be preserved in modern society. The Asian intellectual heritage embraces the whole cycle of life that most of Western psychology has studiously avoided. The practitioner who views his training as merely a means of self-defense will eventually realize that his efforts are unrewarding. The martial Way is nothing less than self-cultivation and the promotion of virtuous conduct. The most important test of a martial artist is always the most difficult one, and that invariably occurs at the most inopportune moment. That is why it is called a "martial art."

When one is threatened or under attack, it is natural to feel fear and anxiety. But fear is not harmful to the spirit of the martial artist. What is damaging to the spirit is either not knowing what to do, or the nagging voice of an external authority. Happy is the individual who trusts his own judgement enough to distinguish reality from illusion and fact from vanity. The Yaqui shaman-sorcerer Don Juan advises:

> "When a man decides what to do, he must go all the way, but he must take responsibility for what he does. No matter what he does, he must know first why he is doing it, and then he must proceed with his actions without having doubts or remorse about them."[1]

The highest form of proficiency in the martial arts is to be able to walk away from a fight without having to fight. Fighting often only perpetuates more fighting; although when confronted with a recurrent evil, there may be no other choice. Like an animal backed into a corner where retreat is no longer possible, it braces itself for the final ultimate confrontation. The true martial artist has enough inner strength and confidence to know that he never has to demonstrate his ability for the sake of showmanship or even to gratify his own ego needs. He knows that, if given no choice, he is prepared to react to an unprovoked attack by mustering all the capabilities within himself. Even if defeated by a more formidable opponent, he might still be able to walk away with his pride intact because he knows that he did everything he could—first to avoid the fight—then to do everything in his power to win it. If he has done his absolute best, then he has passed the test regardless of the outcome of the fight. In certain respects, individuals in modern society need to be faced with life-and-death situations, if only metaphorically. An individual is always capable of going further, doing more than he knows. His potential always exceeds his reach. A man's identity lies in the choice of the possibilities open to him, giving him the power to make sustained acts of choice.

A warrior must be concerned with doing the very best that he can do, limited only by the circumstances beyond his control. Reaching for this ideal easily transcends the parameters of speed or strength. From the master sage to the dedicated *shodan* to the rank novice, there are always those above and below us. It is useless to be envious of another's talents or accomplishments. In practicing the martial arts, the *sifu* can become great by striving for precision; but the middle-aged businessman, the earnest young mother as well as the distracted teenager, all potentially wise as well, can strive for precision—and think of perfection. The reach to develop our heroic nature is worked out in the plain everyday details of our daily lives, and its underlying passion central to a person's individual calling.

The greatest gift of self-proficiency is the relaxed, confident feeling it generates inside. That sense of assurance comes from the knowledge that one has prepared properly, and that everything is under control (to the extent that any situation can be within one's control). Open-minded, clear-headed common sense is the ready position for any confrontation: to think for oneself; to be a leader, not a follower; to not simply mimic the one with the strongest voice or the most authority. The overwhelming majority of those who train diligently in the martial arts never achieve even a modicum of celebrity or wealth, but they do achieve something significant in their own lives. An obscure martial artist is still a true martial artist, and that intrinsically is a great achievement because the meaning lies in the difficulty of the effort itself.

Life is a battle between positive and negative forces. It reflects the oldest and most basic conflict faced by man since the beginning of time—the conflict of good versus evil. The martial artist and the warrior need to believe in the meaningfulness and importance of his actions. He believes in the power of goodness and virtue and its ability to eventually triumph over the forces of evil and darkness. He holds the conviction that, somewhere along the line, what he is and does will make a difference in his actual experience. The warrior exults in the excitement of the battle for a good cause, relishes the joys of victory, and perseveres in the face of defeat. He upholds a faith that his sacrifices will be worth even the ultimate price.

At the same time, there is another battle looming internally, inside his mind. The martial Way may involve fighting with others, but fighting against oneself is the more difficult challenge. During a lifetime, an individual will have many opportunities to overcome his imperfections and amoral tendencies. His human nature will at times turn him to thoughts of desire, fame and profit. These forces threaten to keep him in a cycle of greed, lust and delusion. The average person is all too preoccupied with his cravings for pleasure, wealth and other worldly enjoyments. The vast preponderance of his thinking revolves around his wishes, troubles, and hopes. Such tendencies are an innate part of man's being and are not sinful; but if they remain unchecked, they lead to greed, fear and alienation. If one pursues a virtuous path, worldly success may be a result or by-product to be enjoyed. However, that is all they represent and nothing more.

Without a moral and spiritual context, one cannot attain a lasting, inner peace. That is because happiness cannot be fully defined in terms of wealth, power, fame or even posterity. Knowing this, an individual can push back his concern with possessions and status, and raise his lot in life by consciously making direct choices about who he is, what he has, and what he does. The martial artist who trains with discipline and lives with virtue attains an aura of energy, focus and dominance. He feels it in every fiber of his body, and this kind of power becomes self-evident even to his opponent. When this surge of power occurs, he will overwhelm his opponent. This kind of personal power goes beyond physical strength and technical ability. It is the force of a calm, resolute mind that will not accept fear or failure. Don Juan sums it up this way when he describes how a warrior, as an impeccable hunter who hunts power, becomes a man of knowledge: "For me the world is weird because it is stupendous, awesome, mysterious, unfathomable;... you must assume responsibility for being here, you must learn to make every act count since you are going to be here for only a short while." This is how the warrior "stops the world" and can "see" what is around him. This is how he becomes a "luminous" being.[2]

For each and every person, happiness means using his wealth wisely, knowing that his assets and accomplishments have accumulated without detriment to others, and that he is free of indebtedness to anyone. Knowing that life is finite, the only viable choice is to relish it day by day, moment by moment. Otherwise, at death's door a man may realize too late that he has not made good use of what he has had. When a martial artist practices a *kata* with care, everyone around him knows it; and when he does it carelessly, that is recognized as well even though nothing may be said. When one sits down to take a meal, a cup of tea is as good as a glass of vintage wine even though the latter may seem far more costly and rare. In the memoirs of Gichin Funakoshi, the founder of modern *karate*, he followed some daily habits in his adult life. For example, he awoke early in the morning, dressed and combed his hair, a process that sometimes took an hour. He believed that a samurai must always have an impeccable appearance. Afterwards, he would turn in the direction of the Imperial Palace and bow to the emperor. Only after these rites were completed would he sip his morning tea.

The pursuit of simplicity, of restraint over excess, makes a man more attentive to the beauty of the everyday. In life's thousand and one daily details, seeing the value of one thing or another comes down to a matter of choice. Whether a martial artist is fighting for his life or grooming himself, there are no ordinary moments. If he transforms everything he does into an act of training, then everything he does becomes important. Anything that is important is worthy of his thought, effort and attention. Understanding the difference between knowing and not knowing lets him walk down the path with a peaceful heart. Then he may find that all the power, grace and beauty that he seeks is already within his reach. But he must open his eyes and his mind to see them.

It was Socrates in the West who first taught us that the most important convergence occurs within our selves. This kind of education has many by-products—some good, some bad—all of them disturbing. Only much later does the student know that the "splinter of Socratic irony" has entered his spirit, an occurrence for which he will be always grateful. For the ways in which a person understands the reality of our world are via his mind, body, and spirit. Until all three aspects are integrated, a person is not yet whole and therefore, not fully capable of seeing the whole world. In particular, the convergent capacities of the mind not only determine what one knows but also how one evaluates what one knows. It expands the imagination and engenders clarity of thought and action. The objective is no less than the Socratic ideal of an individual who thinks for himself, uses independent judgement, and acts with deliberate choice. Can a martial artist be virtuous if he feels satisfaction in harming someone else? What good is knowledge of something if that knowledge is not infused with a sense of virtue? Can an immoral person really understand the truth? Can reality be perceived by an unjust mind? Finally and perhaps most importantly, can one really know and believe in something and then fail to implement it? An individual can only contemplate the ideal human character from the perspective of personal transcendence.

There is a deep affinity between personal transformation and the external world. Modern Western philosophy has long proposed the concept that the emergence of reason and order reveals itself gradually through the long dialectic of historical events. In particular, the German philosopher Hegel, in his seminal work *The Phenomenology of Mind* published in 1806, described how the adoption of intellect and organization leads both individuals and societies onto progressively higher forms of spirituality or *geist*. However, the belief that human beings are moving inexorably, if however haphazardly, towards higher forms of consciousness has been seriously challenged by the events of the last hundred years. The skeptics point to the layers of racism, dogmatism and material deprivation that still envelops much of the world. The victims of recurring wars, genocide, disease and ignorance in the twentieth century gave credence to the pessimistic dictum that the dark side of human nature has changed very little over the last 40,000 years. Can we blame them for holding the view that life offers a cyclical or static existence to which time provides very little that is new? For those who care about such questions, which worldview—sustained progress or recurring cyclicality—does one embrace?

Martial arts practice teaches students to take a larger view of life. The fusion of cognition and action is the ultimate test for the martial artist. For the individual, the ultimate convergence is the marriage of a disciplined, physical force and a spiritual, moral force. To be a true martial artist, one must train hard. But one must also be a good citizen, be a good parent, do good deeds, and think good thoughts. It is important and useful to have a powerful punch and a fast kick, but the value of living a virtuous life is the most essential aspect of training. Only then can a martial artist put into practice the Way of goodness and thereby discard the Way of violence and aggression. In Heidegger's terms, the martial arts can increase our power over oneself and others, but it is for naught if a person does not retain a direct connection to humanity, to his relatedness with others. No matter how brilliant and powerful, an individual is but a link in the chain of humanity and cannot exist as an isolated point in time and space. An individual can attain a mastery over other beings but lose the sense of Being itself.

How does the intelligent individual break free from his isolated thinking? How does he maintain a connection with his physical presence and his emotional depth? He can begin by looking at himself as he really is, and examining his strengths and weaknesses, his hopes and illusions, by embracing the Socratic maxim that wisdom begins from an awareness of his own ignorance. He must open his eyes, recognize his strengths and define his objectives. The beginner martial arts student instinctively looks to his *sifu* for answers. He assumes that, with the passage of time and effort, the teacher's knowledge and insights may be transmitted to the student, making him (for better or worse) more like the teacher. This reflexive gravitation towards experts who can deliver solutions reflects human being's myths about certainty and completeness.

In the end, the journey through the martial arts is not about filling in the missing pieces of a complex puzzle. There are precious few secrets or magic tricks. For the advanced student, the parts of the world in which he now travels are mostly empty voids, places without masters, spaces only he can fill. Men for the most part fear the freedom of the unknown, fear being alone. Ultimately he is alone because no one else can understand the things each man feels in his own heart. This higher level of being dictates that each individual finds for himself his own unrevealed destiny in accordance with his desires. The freedom of new beginnings—the pull of what is to be—transforms what may appear to others as aloneness and uncertainty into a daily gift of life. Like Sisyphus in the myth, he finds his universe neither sterile nor futile; in spite of his burdens, he knows himself to be the master of his days.

So there it is, empty space and uncertainty awaits us! The Taoist classic *Chuang Tzu* describes it wonderfully as "being in the realm of Nothing whatever." And the only way these spaces (or the things that we put in these spaces) will have any real meaning will be the ideas and skills that each person works out for himself. All an individual is left with is the freedom to try out what he can do in the face of the "absolute," the "infinite void." As he moves out further along the path of his journey, he finds himself alone again. He has now traveled well beyond the automatic responses and well-worn ruts of his routine world. This is hard to do because from uncertainty arises fear. The experience of Nothing recalls the pristine purity of when he first began to embark on his long life journey.

Over two millennia ago, the ancient Chinese sages already anticipated that the journey of the human spirit in search of freedom and security was destined to be a long and arduous one. Across the expanse of many centuries and disparate cultures, a small number of wise and brave souls steadfastly followed this path, even in the face of persecution, tribalism, gangsterism and brutality. Extending all the way through our modern day, there has been an amazing uniformity of experience on the part of those individuals who listen to the call of the mythical philosopher-warrior-king. In his masterpiece *The Open Society and its Enemies*, the

philosopher Karl Popper tried to disclose to us the sources of man's proclivity to acquiesce to the powers of demagoguery, tribalism, racism and
wanton violence. First published in 1943 war-torn Europe in the midst
of man's single greatest act of catastrophic self-destruction, his concluding sentiments were this:

> *There is no return to a harmonious state of nature.*
> *If we turn back, then we must go the whole way—we*
> *must return to the beasts….. if we shrink from the*
> *task of carrying our cross of humaneness, of reason,*
> *of responsibility, if we lose courage and flinch from*
> *the strain, then we must try to fortify ourselves with*
> *a clear understanding of the simple decision before*
> *us….We must go on into the unknown, the uncer-*
> *tain and insecure, using what reason we may have to*
> *plan as well as we can for both security and free-*
> *dom.*[3]

It is unlikely that Popper, separated by the vast enormity of time and
space, was ever inspired by or was even familiar with *Chuang Tzu*. But
in this context, both the substance and style of these two particular
thinkers resonate to a remarkable degree. For even the truest warrior
finds it daunting to be alone and without companionship. The inadequa-
cy of his knowledge and the inconsistency of his resolve constantly
threaten to turn him away from the chosen path. Someone who
embraces the martial Way has trained to accept the possibility of calami-
ty. He stoically knows that agony and pain, disappointment and torment
are an integral part of life that cannot always be overcome through sheer
effort. By constantly seeking the sources of his own motivations, he will
in time attain the serenity he wishes for. Kierkegaard has described this
type of warrior as "the knight of faith," someone who accepts his lot without complaint, views his responsibilities as a duty, and faces his death
with courage. The knight of faith lives fully in his immediate world and
on his own terms, but places his trust in a higher spiritual dimension.

I have discovered that the Way of the samurai is death. In a fifty-fifty life or death crisis, simply settle it by choosing immediate death. There is nothing complicated about it. Just brace yourself and proceed.

— Tsunetomo Yamamoto (Hagakure)

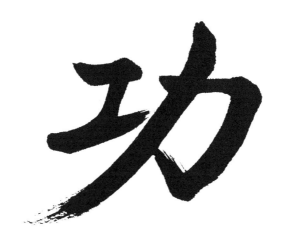

gung
a potent concentration of effort

The Martial Way | II

Through the millennia, man has been subject to aggression and violence from other men, and has pondered ways to meet such hostilities through flight, resistance and counterattack. The quest for the knowledge and skills necessary for self-defense continues to this day. The threat of unprovoked aggression necessitates this quest. As we now plunge headlong into the twenty-first century, recent world events have reminded us of the fragile nature of our civilized society. In fact, acts of terrorism and malevolence have had the unintended effect of making us confront the reality of evil and the personal sacrifices required to defend the values of a modern civilized society. In a world where we face ever-changing threats and increased risks, we need a different kind of security.

The very concepts of self-defense, the martial arts, and a warrior mindset would become irrelevant in the absence of enemies and adversaries in real life. In the empty space just beyond the reach of the fist and the blow of the sword, there is always an opponent staring into our eyes. Abstract ideas do not stare back at us, other human beings do. Whether it is strategy or technique, it is imperative that we must understand the strengths and weaknesses of an opponent in order to defeat him.

The source of man's ceaseless conflict lies in his nature. The philosopher Thomas Hobbes described man's life as "solitary, poor, nasty, brutish and short." Men are just not content with the simple life. They want what they do not yet have and lust enviously for what others possess. They are often greedy, acquisitive and competitive. At times, violence is met in random encounters with unknown assailants in isolated attacks. At other times, displays of brute force are simply the instinctual manifestations of human belligerence and greed. Often such aggression, in the form of tribalism or racism, is initiated by a desire to degrade an external target in order to validate the claims of superiority or uniqueness on the part of the aggressors. This results in the encroachment of territory and the rivalry for limited resources. In the extreme, such aggression leads to organized state warfare. Violent aggression is a state of mind. This proclivity resides in man's psyche; it arises out of fear, ignorance and restlessness.

Men resort to physical force in order to protect their own interests, including the physical security of themselves and their loved ones, their property and their dignity. The late fourteenth-century historical Chinese novel *Three Kingdoms* provides a template for the Asian mentality concerning human relations. It tells of the struggles of three rulers who tried in vain to reunify China in the period 168–265 A.D. The opening lines foretell the recurring themes of power and struggle, loyalty and betrayal, idealism and cynicism in human affairs: "Empires wax and wane; states cleave asunder and coalesce. Thus it has ever been."[4] The essence of human history is conflict. The novel expounds upon the strategy of using deception to triumph against a stronger adversary, if possible, without risking one's own forces.

The act of war is one of the constants of a so-called "civilized society" and seems to be a default state of the human species. Regardless of whether it takes place on an individual or group level, it always refers to the imposition of will by one party over another through subtle or outright violence. Men's endowed instincts, both peaceful and aggressive, have become overlaid with warlike institutions. After five millennia, can our political, economic and technological progress finally produce a stable society? Or will man's fears, self-interest and ignorance irretrievably drag him back into the brutality and bloodshed of history? How many times in history have we seen frustrated individuals, conflicted by their emotions and unbalanced in their physicality, dangerously manipulate other people and events for their own tragic ends? The ideals of the martial arts and martial virtues teach us how to balance our mental and physical skills and to find an awareness of our center. The paradox of finding a balance is the constant deviation from and instinctive realignment with the center of our private lives.

The modern civilized world now promotes many alternatives for conflict resolution in place of overt violence, ironically even as the proliferation of lethal weapons grows exponentially. Consequently, over time the physical strength, mental determination, and emotional endurance necessary for defense of self, family and country have lost their urgency and relevance in today's society. In the post-industrial cyber-culture society we now live in, the traditional male advantages of size and strength are increasingly no longer prerequisites for industry or even defense. The belief held in many cultures that the body is separate from and subordinate to the mind has led to much confusion and suffering. In particular, physical conditioning and muscular development has come to be viewed as unnecessary in modern life. The complacent and sedentary person fails to see the direct correspondence between the spirit and the body: flaccid muscles may reflect feeble emotions, and a paunchy belly indicative of a defeatist mind. Over a century ago, the German philosopher Nietzsche thus anticipated the coming of a generation of self-satisfied "men without chests," preoccupied with their petty worldly wants and lacking any desire for excellence or achievement.[5] A towering product of the Western tradition, like Hegel and Plato before him, Nietzsche believed that men would become soft and self-absorbed in the absence of discipline and sacrifice. In response, he commended martial prowess and stated simply: "The free man is a *warrior*."[6]

Separately, emerging from the East, the martial Way offered an alternative path. The simultaneous training of the mind and the body is one of its central principles. The martial Way offers a different kind of knowledge that cannot be grasped solely through books and direct experience; it must also be grounded in our muscles, blood and bones. This is because embracing the martial Way requires a high level of energy that takes the form of intellectual insight, physical strength, emotional stability and spiritual capacity.

The practice of martial arts, like other physical endeavors grounded in a spiritual tradition, returns us to our own bodies and thus shapes many of our most fundamental attitudes. The correspondence between physical attributes and mental attitudes implies a direct relationship between cardiovascular conditioning and perseverance of will, neuromuscular coordination and emotional poise, body flexibility and open-mindedness, and overall bodily balance and mental stability. The martial artist in training brings his body and mind to the training hall. Relying only upon himself, he focuses his efforts and thoughts in developing his entire being—mind, body and soul—to its highest potential. Ideally, this act requires a total effort of concentration, resolve and calmness of mind. The virtues of martial arts training lies in its simplicity, innocence and call upon the physical, mental, and spiritual dimensions of the practitioner.

The classical martial arts (specifically the fighting arts of unarmed self-defense) which is the subject of this essay, are nearly as old as the history of modern man. Historically, the martial arts sprung directly from the philosophy and religion of Buddhism, without transition from or association with any sport. The historical genesis from Buddhism is explored in greater detail in the following chapter on the evolution of one school of the martial arts. This monumental fact, more than anything else, accounts for the profundity and continuing relevance of the martial Way. The practice of the martial arts is more difficult to convey than just a philosophical idea or a set of techniques. The founder of karate Funakoshi has described the role of karate in modern life this way: "Deep within the shadows of human culture lurk seeds of destruction, just as rain and thunder follow in the wake of fair weather. If a man is overly complacent, trusting that the fair weather will last forever, he will one day be caught off guard...To remember troubled days in days of peace and to constantly train one's body and mind form the guiding spirit and character [of a warrior]."[7] Although the inevitable hostilities between men have historically been the starting points in the origins of the martial arts, the martial way of life has evolved from a practical and necessary means of self-defense in a dangerous world into a broader idealization of how to live the virtuous life. While the martial arts revolve around the art of personal combat, it also demands that its adherents live in accordance with a certain warrior code of conduct and honor.

In the parlance of the martial arts, living the martial Way is a *do* (a way of living), not a *jitsu* (a set of techniques). For those who seek it, the martial Way promises a long and arduous journey. It requires physical effort, mental discipline, and receptivity to values and methods that may strongly counter the ones prevailing in today's world. Entering the world of the martial arts is an invitation to the subordination of self, the endurance of sustained practice, and the cultivation of the body and mind, even in the face of great crisis and fear. It is a highly stoical and austere discipline, with no tolerance for self-indulgences of any kind.

The famous passage quoted at the top of this chapter heading about "choosing immediate death" over life is from *Hagakure* ("hidden in the leaves"), the classic eighteenth-century Japanese primer on samurai ethics and behavior by Tsunetomo Yamamoto. Yamamoto was a samurai whose lord passed away in 1700. Being a loyal retainer, he intended to honor his master by committing *seppuku* or disemboweling himself, but was prevented from doing so by the edicts of the ruling Tokugawa government. Instead, he became a monk and lived out his remaining days in seclusion. He recorded his views on the *bushido* code on scrolls that were later posthumously published.

The *Hagakure* has provided inspiration for generations of warriors who embraced the martial arts as both a secular occupation and a spiritual calling. It later came to the attention of the West during World War II with the stunning advent of the Japanese suicide *kamikaze* pilots who were instructed to crash their bombers into American aircraft carriers. Although the sentiments expressed in *Hagakure* seem extreme to us today, we need to understand that the milieu the samurai lived in was a feudal Japan where warfare and civil strife continued nearly unabated for over three hundred years. In those times, the samurai frequently faced situations where a single, committed stroke of the sword separated life from death. As a result, the classical warrior always prepared himself as if any confrontation would be his last. This impassive attitude did not reflect an indifference to life and death among the samurai class; for the instinct to survive was surely as strong within them as it has always been in all human beings. Ironically, the inspirational purpose of *Hagakure* was to put the contemplation of life against death into a larger perspective.

This preoccupation with death is one that philosophers from antiquity to the present day have used to force a man to truly confront his own nature and the nature of his world. Plato's philosophy is centered on a conscious embrace of death. In his account of the death of Socrates, he explains how a man who has lived philosophically finds the courage to die because the act of philosophy is an exercise in accepting death.[8] The ancient Greek philosophers, the Christian theologians, the Buddhists and Taoists, and the modern day existentialists all shared the notion that death must be contemplated in order to appreciate life. Kierkegaard, in a key passage from *Concluding Unscientific Postscript* thus wrote:

> *We wish to know how the conception of death will transform a man's entire life, when in order to think its uncertainty he has to think of it in every moment, so as to prepare himself for it.*[9]

The fear and anxiety of death is misguided because people have difficulty accepting the fact that they are going to die. In the native American culture, the Yaqui Indian Don Juan continues this long philosophical tradition when he describes death in an embodied form—death as an advisor:

> *Death is our eternal companion. It is always to our left, at an arm's length….It has always been watching you. It always will until the day it taps you. Death is the only wise advisor that we have.*[10]

Because it so concentrates the mind, it is in the face of death that we see our lives most clearly. In our busy everyday life, it is only too convenient to avoid facing the most basic questions: How should we live? What are our strengths and weaknesses? What is most precious to us? For too many people, it requires the prospect or threat of death to examine these questions. Thus Heidegger in *Being and Time* wrote that for the great majority of human beings, this question of being "will strike but once like a muffled bell that rings into our life and gradually dies away."[11] Heidegger returned philosophical inquiry to its proper foundations by directing it back to the actual conditions of a human life in the natural and social world.

Philosophers of all ages exist to remind us of what man's purpose in life should be. They plant the notion in an individual's mind that perhaps something essential is missing, and then compels him on a mysterious journey. Such a journey may take the traveler to the depths of an abyss or to the dizzying heights of a vertical ascent. A man should feel at all times that there are important things for which he lives; and even his death will not put an end to these interests that will survive him. But no matter how much the armchair philosopher contemplates the idea of death, as long as he fails to attain the physical courage to ever face it, he cannot truly grasp the concept. In its appeal to the heroic side of our nature, the martial Way provides us with an answer to these essential questions. Through martial arts training, we mobilize the *gung*, the highly focused and potent concentration of effort, which is the mental and spiritual foundation of all the martial arts.

Martial arts training is deadly serious, literally a matter of life and death. In any confrontation with an opponent, the true martial artist must act as if one blow determines everything. If a mistake is made, he will fall. The martial arts involve both physical training and mental conditioning. The devotee must train himself both physically and mentally; therefore mental discipline is both a precondition of learning the art and also the result of undergoing such training. The martial artist who has trained properly over time is a confident, tranquil person. An economy of movement characterizes his actions. Even in the midst of chaos and fear, there is no posturing or chattering. This cultivated persona is all the more deceptive because it masks the martial arts' traditional lethal nature, calling upon the capacity to maim or kill using one's own hands.

The experienced martial artist grasps the seriousness of his practice. He knows of the real possibility of inflicting harm on someone else, or of being harmed himself. The most lethal aspects of the martial arts are rarely obvious to the casual observer because the principle of calm appearance masking underlying strength is always at work. Therefore, the martial artist must always consider how far he is willing to go in the actual use of his hard-earned skills, and that ethos is an integral part of his spiritual training.

In feudal Japan, the samurai had the legal right to kill a commoner who showed him disrespect, but his sense of honor and restraint embodied in the warrior's *bushido* code made this kind of occurrence rare. To control the power of his martial training, he must first control himself. The student who studies the art only in order to fight rarely continues training for very long. Only those with a higher ideal will find the art compelling enough to persevere in its training. In developing inner strength and balance, he must train his spirit as he would train his body, confronting the essential matters of life and death. Martial arts without compassion and honor promises only violence. Stripped of its spirituality, it threatens injury and suffering to both its victims and its practitioners. In the end, this higher ideal is what separates the warrior from the predator.

In modern times, we do not typically face life and death as part of our everyday routine. Nevertheless, the meaning of life and death, and living in accordance with its implications, lies at the heart of following the martial Way. This is because those who have experienced brushes with death or have been in life-threatening situations are privileged to have a certain perspective not readily available to most other people. Such near-death experiences often change their attitudes and behaviors, at least for a period of time before habitual patterns of thinking reassert themselves. In this light, what might be previously thought of as acts of heroism, sacrifice or great effort would be otherwise transformed into something trivial. The relationships that are formed with others, and one's very self-perceptions, take on a much more profound and lasting meaning when a human life lies in the balance. The realization of impending death shocks a man to his core and reduces his world to its most elemental components—the kind of world philosophers and theologians speak of. The typical complaints, irritations and regrets of daily life quickly reveal themselves as petty self-indulgences, not real problems. The specter of death also forces men out of their own private egos, reminding them that they belong to something larger than themselves. It is the consciousness of death that dignifies life.

The common term for the place where martial arts training occurs is the familiar but misunderstood Japanese word *dojo* or the traditional training hall (literally, the place to practice the way.) The lesser known Chinese counterpart is the term *gwan* or *kwoon*. Much more than simply referring to a school or a physical place, the *dojo* broadly represents the methodological, philosophical and spiritual dimensions of martial arts training. It is both a physical place as well as a state of mind. The spirit of a *dojo*, as exemplified by its *sifu* or *sensei*, instructors and students, is built on the ideal of warrior virtue. Every member of this community works toward the achievement of a virtuous life by the attainment, in part, of a mastery of self-defense techniques. We train because it is a part of our life, and we do it for its own sake. The skills and knowledge that we acquire must fit into our life and be consistent with the values that we embrace.

The formulation of a new way of thinking and acting begins with the expression of a variety of forms to capture a single, perhaps still ambiguous theme. In time, only when the right combination of training, experience and insight come together does that theme becomes a part of oneself. Achieving proficiency in the martial arts requires the acquisition of skills, prolonged training, and an extensive understanding of oneself and one's opponents. To understand and practice one's own chosen style is the starting point. Over a long period of time, this may lead to an awareness of the interconnectedness of other martial arts styles, and ultimately, to an understanding of how we relate to others in our world.

The essence of all martial arts transcends a mere physical confrontation between two belligerents. Instead, it is a vehicle for the martial artist to reach towards inner peace, self-confidence, and ultimately, the unification of mind and body. But the progression towards these goals is neither predictable nor linear. Often there are long plateaus in which true progress seems to stop for extended periods of time. Occasionally, the practitioner may even reverse course due to frustration or negligence, until some new insight leads him back to the right way. At times, we all ask ourselves why we have stopped progressing? We question the apparent meaninglessness and tedium of continuing practice. In periods of disappointment and frustration, we wonder why the practice of martial arts is so demanding and difficult.

After a while, even the most devoted martial artist realizes that it often is not possible to make rapid progress. True progress is always little by little, repeating something over and over again. In these moments of discouragement, it is critical to remember that frustrations and setbacks are an unwelcome but central part of martial arts practice. Just as in life when we cannot select the foe with whom we choose to do battle, so it is the same in training. Whether it is in the artificiality of the *dojo* or the rough-and-tumble of the street, the martial artist passes each day responding to adversity as it arises. The benefit of sustained practice is the enhanced ability to respond flexibly to all kinds of critical confrontations. He utilizes his skills and his power to continue down this path. He does not have the luxury of clear skies, good health and a sunny disposition whenever he needs it. Instead, he must sometimes persevere through fatigue, pain and self-doubt at the most inauspicious times. That is what makes martial arts training so difficult at times.

The martial Way does not offer a linear or even one-dimensional path toward progress. The process more closely resembles a spherical and uneven ascent. True proficiency can be achieved only after a prolonged period of application and commitment. Month after month, year after year, our martial arts experience will deepen until it encompasses all aspects of our everyday life. When we know, in our heart of hearts, that we have gone to the limits of our physical and mental abilities, there is an inner calm. This calm arises from the knowledge that, even in the face of great anxiety, we are able to make rational decisions about which options to choose. This calm extends to all aspects of personal life, far beyond the *dojo*. Personal serenity engenders greater tolerance when dealing with others, patience in working towards our objectives, and graciousness in accepting life's inevitable setbacks.

The circularity of the martial arts is what makes it so challenging, and seem so esoteric. Every martial arts style, no matter how complex, has a limited number of techniques and strategies to learn. Once the serious student has gained some proficiency in a given system, he has literally traversed a great circle only to end up where he began. Instead of learning yet another technique, he now needs to master what he has already learned. In time, he will find that the most important secrets and subtleties of his art lie in the most fundamental and simple techniques and concepts. Only in retrospect can the veteran black belt know that the "secrets" he wanted so desperately to learn were already contained during his white belt training. He just could not see it at the beginning of his training. The concept of personal progress and time, circling within itself and repeating a limited repertoire, is a well-established tradition in Eastern thought.

Paradoxically, embracing the martial Way (outside of the training hall) involves little ritual or ceremony because the process and the hope of enlightenment are decidedly personal. On the surface, it does not require a dramatic change in behavior, but rather the attainment of an understanding of the nature of everyday life. The development and maturation of a martial artist involves a long, slow and subtle process. Taking the first step in this journey of knowledge, the novice learns the beginner's techniques, trains for a long period of time, confronts doubts and disappointments, and gradually is guided by his teacher to a higher level of realization. At the end, he discovers that he may still be at the beginning, that the first technique is also the last, that he still must practice every day, and that the greatest virtue lies in the pursuit of simplicity.

Modern martial arts philosophy in regards to confrontation and violence, though remaining grounded in pacifism and evasion of conflict, has taken a more pragmatic turn. The very act of confrontation implies facing up to an adversary. If a warrior is moral, just, and can empathize with his fellow man, then his enemy likely dwells in the shadow of evil. In this regard, the human record has shown that men are beyond redemption. There is evil in the world. No matter how much a man struggles to uphold what is right, the injustices and sufferings in this world will always remain. That evil exists and accumulates in the minds of men is beyond the shadow of a doubt. The turning points in history are always ignited by the persistent encroachments of evil over good. Humane values and lofty intentions cannot prevail unless they are enforced by the power of the sword and the force of righteous will. As one political journalist has noted, in surveying both the secular and the spiritual realm of man, "only armed prophets succeed."[12] Accordingly, the martial artist knows the foolishness of unnecessary combat, but he must also know the wisdom of necessary resistance. Although the warrior's credo is always to find a reasonable means to avoid fighting, it is balanced by his ability and willingness to do battle. Except for those who have renounced living in the everyday world, circumstances abound when it is both right and necessary to defend oneself against aggression. Pacifism cannot be sustained without martial readiness.

It is axiomatic that a successful action is derived from a sense of self-confidence. The person who is alert and confident is also the most likely one to deter the possibility of attack from hostile sources. Thus, the warrior's sword may be drawn but it does not leave the scabbard unless it is ready to be used. The warrior resorts to his weapons sparingly, and when he does he is swift, moving away without leaving a trace. It is not a matter of bravery or cowardice. In the face of evil and cruelty, he knows he must stand up in defense of what is worth protecting. Albert Camus, in his meditation on the rebel and necessary resistance, describes it beautifully this way: "At this moment, when each of us must fit an arrow to his bow… the bow bends, the wood complains. At the moment of supreme tension, there will leap into flight an unswerving arrow, a shaft that is inflexible and free."[13] The warrior never cowers before evildoers. He chooses to fight back and resists becoming a victim. To acquiesce to unbridled aggression only invites disaster and threatens all that which he holds dear. To stay with the same metaphor, Eugen Herrigel in *Zen In the Art of Archery* describes eloquently exactly who should fit the arrow to the bow, when it should be released, and how the arrow finds its target. He describes how the bow and the archer eventually becomes one. In a similar vein, we idealize that the warriors of both antiquity and today represent the thorns on a rose, guarding what is beautiful yet vulnerable.

Under such circumstances, the warrior knows that victory will belong to him no matter what the outcome. When he encounters a true opponent, even one who is superior in strength and skill, if he cannot avoid the fight, then he must make his stand. That is what makes the martial artist also a warrior. The power that a martial artist acquires is a feeling or a mood. He understands the source of this power because he can sneak in between the world of ordinary people and the world of warriors, and can contemplate the glory of victory with the agony of defeat. He believes that such power can be stored and available for use when he needs it. The warrior is a fighter and a man of action. He takes an aggressive, alert stance towards the world. He trains his mind and body, is ready to face both life and death, and embraces a transcendent value beyond himself.

As a result, he faces the world with both a sense of detachment as well as an attitude of active engagement. The detachment is necessary because the warrior needs both mental and physical separation from his adversaries in order to act forcefully. When he uses lethal force to subdue his enemies, it is only in order to protect the good and the vulnerable from the clutches of bullies and predators. By truthfully following the path of a warrior, he endures the hardships of learning, and without either rushing or faltering, goes as far as he can go in unraveling the secrets of his personal power. But it is a form of power expressed through strength and compassion. When he embraces this idea, his world itself changes.

This concept of power as the cornerstone of personal freedom lies at the bottom of all martial arts philosophy. The recognition that power emanates from physical force and martial capability cuts both ways; it can be channeled towards constructive uses or abused as a means of destruction. This is the reason why martial arts training must always been directed towards the cultivation of the higher ideals of discipline, humility, benevolence and responsibility.

In the modern day, the dedicated martial artist practices his art as a way to pursue self-mastery. He embraces the traditional warrior virtues of courage, discipline, integrity, accountability and respect for human life. He does not equate his efforts with winning or losing although he knows that life will present him with many tests over time. Finally, beyond physical training, he cultivates an inner freedom in his own spiritual life that transcends everyday appearances and common materialistic desires. He endeavors to live fully every minute of his life. Whether it is the traditional warrior training of a bygone age or the formal martial arts training which is the subject of this essay, the result is a powerful but peaceful state of consciousness.

Kensho Furuya, the *aikido* master and Zen priest, has summarized it this way: "Hide all your talents, work hard until you die, give everything you have to others, believe in God or Buddha or whoever you follow, and bear all hardships and obstacles patiently and with nobility. This is the life of a true warrior."[14] This state of mind is what gives a man both the physical courage and the moral strength to face the prospect of death in a heroic manner. The martial Way clarifies the nature of both violence and resistance, while providing the body and spirit with the means to pursue self-perfection.

I come to you with only empty hands. I have no weapons, but should I be forced to defend myself, my principles or my honor, should it be a matter of life and death, or right or wrong; then here are my weapons, my empty hands.

—Ed Parker

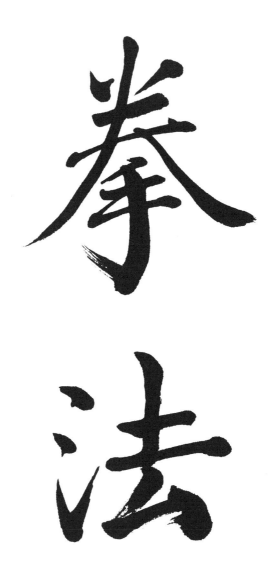

chuan fa (Chn.) / kenpo (Jap.)
law of the fist

China Hand, Empty Hand | III

The following historical discussion of the development of martial arts in Asia focuses on one important strand—a martial arts style known today in the West as *kenpo karate*, from its origins in the Shaolin Temple in China, through its long evolution in Japan, to its importation to the West. While there are, of course, numerous other martial arts styles that have developed in other countries during the last several hundred years, there are few competing martial arts styles of comparable longevity that have been in continuous practice. Moreover, *kenpo* is virtually unique among the major martial arts styles in that its substantive historical development is based on both the Chinese and the Japanese martial arts heritage, drawing from the Shaolin martial arts tradition and the significant contributions of Japanese *jujitsu* and *karate*. The purpose of this discussion, (see Bibliography) is not to give any comparative analysis of *kenpo* relative to other existing schools, rather only to give the reader a historical perspective of one significant martial arts style.

It is the author's belief that no individual martial arts style is inherently superior to another. Petty arguments about the effectiveness and authenticity of rival martial arts styles only serve to diminish the stature of those who have devoted themselves to the martial Way. What matters is the degree to which a martial artist has faith in and can master his chosen style of martial art.

Historical analyses of the martial arts have always been difficult and problematic for historians. This is because the martial arts have long relied upon an oral tradition in the transmission of knowledge from master to disciple. The art was practiced and taught under the utmost secrecy. Much of the details and so-called "secrets" of individual styles were carefully hidden and obfuscated to prevent outsiders from learning too much. In particular, there has been a long-standing bias against the full conveyance of information to Western practitioners. Native martial arts masters had no desire to pass on their precious legacy to strangers who could not appreciate what it truly represented.

For example, George Dillman, one of the most respected martial arts technicians in the United States, has recounted how he discovered for himself that much of what he was taught over four decades of training in the Japanese martial arts represented deliberate misinformation. He eloquently describes the situation this way:

> [The martial arts] can be compared to a song. The meaning of the song is stated in the lyrics and expressed in the melody. If the lyrics are sad, the melody is haunting; if the lyrics are noble, the melody is bold....But what if the lyrics are in a foreign language? Without knowing the meaning of the words, how is it possible to truly comprehend the song?
> For most students of the martial arts, [it] is a song whose lyrics have not been explained. They can appreciate its beauty and power. They have a feel for its rhythms and dynamics. They may even catch some vague sense of its purpose, but without understanding the actual application of the techniques, they cannot truly comprehend the fullness of meaning.[15]

Regrettably, large portions of the Asian martial arts heritage have been handed down to us via legends, anecdotal evidence, and outright myth.

Nevertheless, there is now virtual universal agreement among historians that the history of the martial arts had its origins dating back to the introduction of Buddhism in China. Around 525 A.D., the Indian prince Bodhidharma or Daruma traveled from India to China to spread the teachings of Buddhism. After visiting the imperial court, he eventually traveled to Hunan Province in north central China and settled near the Shaolin Temple. There he found the monks victimized by local robbers, and too thin and weak to defend themselves or pursue their studies. Bodhidharma advised them that war and violence was not a "right action," but it was also wrong not to be in good physical health or to be prepared to defend oneself. Subsequently, he taught them a series of exercises and physical movements (called the 18 Hands of the Lo Han or the "enlightened one") to strengthen their bodies and enhance their mental acuity. Bodhidharma emphasized the development of chi or the body's essential energy source as the crucial dimension of his exercises. For without it, a martial system would merely be physical motion, without any mental mastery. These exercises became the core of Shaolin chuan fa, literally meaning "law of the fist" (better known today as wu shu in China or kung fu in the West), an empty-handed martial art that is the basis from which most of the fighting styles of Chinese, Japanese and Korean martial arts later evolved.

The essence of Bodhidharma's martial arts teachings was subsequently refined and expanded by succeeding Buddhist monks. By this time, Shaolin *chuan fa* had expanded to an art comprised of 170 techniques, many of which were inspired by the five original animal forms (dragon, tiger, crane, snake and leopard) studied by the Shaolin monks. The monks imitated the creatures of nature to develop their bodies and discipline their minds. They tried to distill in their movements the power and tenacity of the tiger, the subtlety and endurance of the snake, the speed and patience of the leopard, the grace and control of the crane, and the passion and fire of the winged dragon. Their goal was to achieve a harmony of mind and body by distilling the virtues of these various animal traits. The monks were drawn to this Shaolin system because of its pacifist philosophical foundation, graceful form and grounding in physical technique.

The practice and dissemination of *wu shing chuan* or "five animal form" set a new stage in the evolution of the martial arts. This form of *chuan fa* subsequently developed in China for over 700 hundred years and eventually spawned hundreds of idiosyncratic and highly specialized fighting styles such as the tiger claw, eagle claw, white crane and praying mantis systems that have persisted through to modern times. For example, *fu-jow pai* (tiger claw system), as the name indicates, was modeled on the spirit and fighting techniques of the tiger. The tiger is a symbol of nobility and recognized for its fierce power and fighting spirit. Once the tiger engages in combat, its commitment is total and irrevocable, fighting to the death if necessary.

During the Tang Dynasty (618-907 A.D.), imperial court records indicated that Japanese Buddhist monks had visited China where they gained some exposure to Shaolin *chuan fa* and subsequently brought this knowledge back to Japan. The introduction of Zen Buddhism to Japan accelerated the transmission of the Chinese fighting arts to the island kingdom. In 1215 A.D., the Japanese monk Eisai returned from China and established the *Rinzai* sect of Zen which relied heavily on the use of Zen *koans* (riddles with no logical answer) to achieve *satori* or spontaneous enlightenment. Shortly thereafter, Eisai's disciple Dogen, in 1253, founded the second major Zen sect, *Soto* Zen that focused on the use of meditation to achieve *satori*.

In the midst of these seminal historical developments, the destiny of Shaolin *chuan fa* also took a decisive turn. Around the time of 1235 A.D. when the Mongol hordes were completing their conquest of China, the head priest of the Shaolin Temple escaped to Japan and sought refuge with a prominent Shinto priest named Kosho at the Shakain Temple in

Kumamoto, on the southern island of Kyshu in Japan. Kosho was already a master in many of the Japanese fighting arts including swordsmanship, archery and an indigenous unarmed fighting art, when he began his study of the *chuan fa* system with the Shaolin high priest. After years of study, Kosho then combined these various fighting systems and attracted a student following in what became known as *koshoryu kenpo* (literally, "old pine tree style fist law"). Later on in life, Kosho changed his family name to Yoshida. At this historical juncture, a crucial aspect of the legacy of Shaolin *chuan fa* was transferred to the Japanese who pronounced the original Chinese *chuan fa* characters as "*kenpo*," referring to it as "Chinese boxing."

In 1280, the Yoshida (Kosho) clan converted to Buddhism and sought to reconcile the lethal warrior-like nature of their martial arts style with the peaceful, passive teachings of Buddha. They espoused the concept of self-defense only as a response to external aggression, and emphasized techniques of escape from attackers with a minimum amount of physical contact. Since the true martial artist valued peace and harmony above victory, their philosophy emphasized avoidance of confrontation. But if avoidance was impossible, then the preferred method of response was not to stop force but to redirect it, back against the aggressor if necessary.

For over 650 years, the *koshoryu kenpo* system, modified from Chinese *chuan fa*, was subsequently passed from generation to generation and taught to members of the extended Yoshida clan and their associates in the samurai class.[16] Historical records document further visits by Ming Dynasty (1368—1644 A.D.) martial arts masters to Japan, via the growing trade between Fukien Province in southern China and Okinawa, during the sixteenth and seventeenth century. During this time, as Shaolin *chuan fa* and its subsequent variations continued to spread throughout China, ongoing travel and exchange between the Chinese mainland, Okinawa and Japan also led to the ongoing modification of *koshoryu kenpo* in Japan. In both countries, however, the teaching of these unarmed fighting styles largely took place within the restricted confines of Buddhist temples and feudal castles, and was strictly off-limits to the general public. Moreover, the practice of any form of martial arts (as well as the possession of weapons) was strictly forbidden by the Japanese government in Okinawa, under the threat of reprisal by armed samurai.

In feudal Japan, warriors had long practiced a system of attack involving throwing, hitting and twisting limbs referred to as *jujitsu* (the "gentle art"). In 1882, the educator Jigoro Kano systematically revised this traditional fighting system and established *judo* (the "gentle Way"), based upon the guiding principal of initially yielding in order to obtain ultimate victory. Shortly thereafter in 1903, *karate* also became known to the public when the Japanese government pressured its leading practitioners to introduce the art into the public school curriculum. This was the catalyst for a veritable renaissance in Japanese martial arts forms. For by the beginning of the twentieth century, thousands of students sought training in *judo* at Jigoro Kano's Kodokan in Tokyo; and in 1920, Morihei Ueshiba established his *aikido* academy near Kyoto.

In 1923, the 21st lineal descendent of the Yoshida clan was born in Hawaii and christened James Masayoshi Mitose. At the age of five, he was repatriated back to Japan and received his religious and martial arts training from his *kenpo* master uncle in the family's Buddhist temple on Mt. Akenkai in southern Japan. For fifteen years, he studied his family's traditional fighting art. Upon his travels, he discovered that the local police had no effective weapons to use in defending the citizenry from bandits and gangsters, and began to teach outsiders *koshoryu kenpo* for the first time. During this period, *karate* was being widely popularized by its founder Gichin Funakoshi in Okinawa. Despite some significant differences in approach between the two martial arts styles, the substantial overlap between *kenpo* and *karate* was self-evident. In fact, the very term *karate* originally denoted the words "China hand;" it was only later in 1933 that the character for "*kara*" (or "*Tang* 唐" meaning China) was replaced by Funakoshi with its homonym "*kara* 空" (meaning "empty"). This significant alteration in the meaning of the word "*karate*" not only suited the pressures of Japanese chauvinism at the time, but also reflected the prevalent anti-Chinese sentiment in militarist Japan. As we will discuss later, this was more than a mere semantic change; for language not only changes the perception of reality, but sometimes reality itself.

In the 1930s, as Japan was poised for war against both China and the United States, Mitose opposed the belligerent policies of the Japanese government and consequently returned to Hawaii in 1936. He established the Honolulu Official Self-Defense Club and began accepting students. From that time until 1956 when Mitose moved to California, he taught *koshoryu kenpo*, first to U.S. Army cadets and later to students of all backgrounds. In 1947, he published the first book in English on the philosophy and techniques of *kenpo* entitled *What Is Self-Defense? (Kenpo Jiujitsu)*.

During the years that Mitose taught *kenpo* in Hawaii, he awarded the *shodan* or first-degree black belt rank to six students. One of them was William Chow who had previously been studying the Chinese *kung fu* martial arts styles. Chow, in turn, opened his own school in the 1949, and began to emphasize many of the circular techniques of *kung fu* as well as its various *kata* or forms. One of William Chow's most prominent students was Edmund Parker, a native Hawaiian who earned his black belt from Chow in 1954 and later immigrated to California. Starting in 1957, it was from Ed Parker's martial arts school in Pasadena, California where the *kenpo* tradition has been spread throughout the United States. In 1964, Ed Parker sponsored the first national martial arts tournament in the United States which was highlighted by the introduction of a then unknown Chinese martial artist from Hong Kong named Bruce Lee. In the 1960s, Ed Parker, along with Bruce Lee (who went on to fame developing his own martial arts style), were arguably the most prominent practicing martial artists in the West. In fact, until Bruce Lee came to international prominence, Chinese *kung fu* styles were virtually unknown in the Western world.

There is now little doubt that the very old system of Shaolin *chuan fa* originated by Boddhidharma was imported to Japan and merged with the indigenous unarmed fighting style of Okinawa in the early decades of the twentieth century to form what is now *chuan fa tang so* (literally "fist law China hand") or better known in the West as *kenpo karate*. The modern *kenpo* system today incorporates many of the kicks of the northern Chinese martial arts styles and the hand strikes of the southern Chinese styles. Specifically, it incorporates the "five animal form" techniques and the Chinese art of joint locks known as *chin na*. Moreover, because of its long evolution in Japan, *kenpo* also incorporates many features of the Japanese systems of *jujitsu* and *karate*. The result is that *kenpo* has emerged from its long historical evolution as a martial arts fighting style grounded in its Chinese Shaolin roots but profoundly influenced by the Japanese samurai *bushido* traditions.

As practiced today, *kenpo* is one of the most lethal martial arts, replete with blocks, kicks, punches joint locks and breaks, and nerve strikes. It is an eclectic fighting system full of hard offensive and soft defensive techniques, characterized by both circular and linear movements. The style emphasizes a continuous flow of motion wherein every move creates a specific reaction in the opponent, and every reaction leads to the next move. Thus every strike is a block; every block is a strike; and each move flows into the next. A clawing hand is followed by a thrust kick, a joint lock is followed by a hip throw, and an evasive block turns into a lethal choke. Although many splinter groups subsequently formed out of Ed Parker's schools during the last three decades, the vast majority of the *kenpo* black belts in the Americas have been awarded by Parker and his expanding circle of followers.[17] It is now widely acknowledged by martial arts historians that the Parker legacy, as continued by his associates since his death in 1990, has been responsible for propagating the *kenpo* tradition in the Western world.

PART II

The Way is in training…
Do nothing which is not of value.
　　　　　　　— Miyamoto Musashi

The famous kendo master was meditating alone in the dojo when his new student called upon him. Waiting until no others were in sight, he anxiously asked the master: "What is the secret of your mastery of the sword?" The master made no movement. After a moment, the student repeated his question whereupon the master instantly grabbed a nearby staff and hit the student on the head with all his might, sending the student head long across the dojo. The master said: "That is my answer."
　　　　　　　— A Zen koan

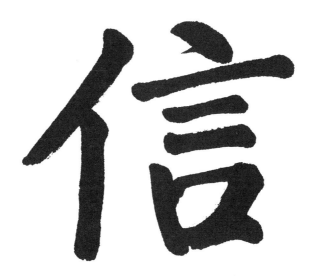

shin
faith

No Magic Wand | IV

When I was a young man and still not yet out of school, I spent a summer as a "Student Work-Scholar" at Esalen Institute in Big Sur, California. In the early 1970s, Esalen was still in its years of resplendent glory, widely recognized as the worldwide mecca for teachers and students interested in the "human potential" movement. Once home to a Native American tribe known as the Esselin, and nestled on a cliff between the Big Sur coastline and the Santa Lucia Mountains rising sharply behind, this magnificent facility hosted ongoing seminars and classes in virtually all the psychotherapies and holistic philosophies in vogue during that period. Seminarians from all over the world flocked to this 27 acres of spectacular California coastline to partake in the classes, the natural hot springs, and the rarefied spiritual aura of this magical place.

In return for participating in the seminars and living on the grounds, I was required to perform various daily tasks such as working in the garden, cleaning the rooms and helping in the office. One of my very first assignments was to clean all the windows in a large, old Victorian house on the grounds. Looking out on the Pacific Ocean, I spent several hours cleaning windows. As I moved into the kitchen, I noticed a small sign taped on the wall on top of the sink. In simple block letters, it read: "Zen masters wash their own bowls." The sink was spotless, and the cleaned dishes were neatly stacked in the dish rack. I pondered that notion and proceeded in my work.

Two aspects of that memory stayed with me. First, to achieve true spiritual enlightenment is to be in elite company, but even the elite is not above the mundane and tedious responsibilities of everyday life. This is why a sense of humility is so central to following the righteous path. Second, even those most preoccupied with matters of the spirit and intellect must also involve themselves equally with matters of the body and the physical world. This balance is inherent in living the martial Way.

These days, many aspiring young martial artists are looking for the secrets that will help them quickly learn the mastery of their art. Dave Lowry, one of the most articulate critics of the commercialism of modern martial arts captures this mood perfectly when he writes: "If I may paraphrase Churchill, never have so many wished for so much while expending so little."[18] Many of today's impatient students seek short cuts to accelerate the arduous and tedious aspects of their chosen style. However, the so-called secrets and subtleties of the art are complex and require time to comprehend. This type of learning does not occur within the framework of weeks and months, but years. Even if the instructor tells the student all the answers, he cannot absorb it in a finite period of time. The naïve student cannot expect to distort, pervert and dilute the art in order to fit it into his own narrow, egotistical conception of time. He cannot apply conventional measures of time and efficiency to a pursuit as important as the martial arts. In a way, the passage of time is in itself a test for the serious student, one that many students will eventually fail.

By casting aside impatience and self-complacency, the dedicated martial arts practitioner knows that he can never be good enough. The moment he believes that he is, then he has stopped learning and thus has stopped living as a true martial artist. For those who persevere in regular training, the martial Way gradually becomes a part of everyday life. In time and with the proper spirit, the true learning of techniques will emerge, on their own. In daily training, it may sometimes seem as if new obstacles are placed in our path constantly. Rarely does everything proceed as planned or without unexpected problems. Yet the martial arts student needs to be reminded that this state of affairs represent the real world in which he lives. A life without setbacks, failures, regrets and sickness is not a real life. These negative developments are as real as everything else in life.

Instead of cynicism or resignation, he must plod on. It means that he needs to be more persistent, resourceful and hopeful from one day to the next. It means that he must enhance his sensitivity and pay greater attention to the details. Though he may never face disaster or the catastrophe of total loss, if he can steel himself against the idea of everything going against us, then that is a starting point from which to focus his energy and devotion to his objectives. Maintaining balance in the face of imminent total loss is truly a worthy victory, a magic wand to help us in our struggles and confrontations.

The demands of work, family, finances, as well as fatigue, neglect and health all distract the martial artist from his best intentions. Even the devoted student may be disappointed if he expects martial arts training to neatly bring his physical and spiritual condition into working order.

Nevertheless, regular training can serve as a constant, to discipline him to develop his best self even as the daily routine pulls him in different directions. The strategies underlying training can be effectively applied not just in life threatening situations but to daily life.

The actual practice of training may be different from the ideal of training. Actual practice is simply doing the same thing again and again, day after day, hoping to become just a little bit better. The student tries to increase his physical power, breathing, muscular flexibility and body coordination. Sometimes he fails to understand the point of it, as he stands in his own sweat and fatigue. Sometimes he makes mistakes and experience injury or discouragement. Students all sometimes ask themselves why they spend so much time on something that has so little apparent practical value. Finally, some are tempted simply to quit.

The martial Way reminds the faithful student to stay on the daily path of practice, to keep his mind fresh and alert, and continue to continue. If he does so, he can approach perfection as a person, with a heightened sensitivity about his mind, body and environment, and an enhanced capacity to deal with the challenges of every aspect of life. Through training, life's hurdles may reveal themselves as our most important teachings. But the powers that are gained, and the lessons learned are highly personal in nature and should be used prudently. In fact, devoted training gives each person a secret power, one that cannot be thoughtlessly revealed. To defeat opponents but to not meet the requirements of daily life indicates a misunderstanding of essential skills.

Maintain your vision while doing your work.
Keep dominion over your desires and attain perfec-
tion.

—Lao Tzu

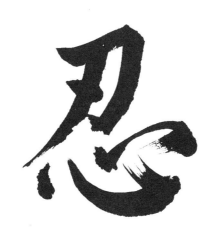

ren (Chn.) / nin (Jap.)
to endure

Practice Real Life | V

Martial arts training involves both a physical and psychological process in which the martial artist becomes conditioned to respond to a potentially threatening situation. One objective of physical training is to develop muscle strength, increase aerobic capacity, and enhance the balance of the nervous system. But the response that is called for is not only a neuromuscular one but also an attitudinal one. It requires the coming together of the body and the mind in such a way as to evade a physical threat, and then to deliver a physical retaliation. Training begins with the conditioning of one's own body. Any possible transformation of self must begin there. One major objective of martial arts training is to prepare students for real-life confrontations. Students sometimes lose sight of this when they concentrate on achieving belt rankings and the practice of forms.

When the student enters the *dojo*, he has nothing to offer except the willingness to do everything that he is told to do. At the beginning of training, he hangs on to the instructor's every word. The apt description for the beginning student might be summarized as follows: "don't ask, don't think, just do!" Like a child, he begins to learn some basic skills. He sees in the instructor a standard towards which he tries to reach. In time, each student finds different methods of improving his abilities. Eventually, through trial and error, experience and insight, serious students find a way for the martial arts to become embedded in the fabric of their daily lives. This happens within the day-to-day mundane routines of practice. As the student learns the art, he gradually executes his movements with more precision, his techniques with more fluidity, and his tactics with more comprehension. If he truly make progress, then the barriers between a martial artist's daily training and his life imperceptibly fade away. So ironically, the traditional martial artist no longer concentrates on his training. He simply lives his life in accordance with a set of values and priorities.

There is a famous Taoist maxim attributable to Chuang-tzu: *"zwo jin guan tien,"* which is translated as "sitting in a well peering up at the sky." It relates to the parable of a frog that dwells at the bottom of a well and has never come up to see the world around it. The frog passes a self-satisfied existence, master of its own domain, glancing only occasionally upwards at the changing vista of the sky through the small opening of the well that is situated on a farm. One day when curiosity finally beckons it to climb out of the well, it encounters for the first time an overwhelming abundance of circumstances and other life forms never imagined before. The frog is simultaneously fascinated and terrified by this much larger and more complex world. As time passes, the frog must decide whether it should return to the secure and simple world that it knew at the bottom of the well, or remain permanently above ground in its newly discovered world. This parable speaks to all those who come to a fork in the road: whether to take the safe and known path, even if it is dull and insignificant; or take an alternate, open path that may lead to something more fulfilling but also more uncertain.

The freedom to choose a path at this fork in the road recalls Plato's famous allegory of the cave. A man who has long been chained in a gloomy cavern is suddenly freed and looks out at the light. But because of the dazzle and the sparkle, he is "unable to discern the objects whose shadows he formerly saw." Likewise, the beginning martial arts student will encounter this choice in his training. In fact, if he perseveres in the journey, he will be confronted with numerous such forks in the road whereupon he must decide whether to jump back in the safe, dark well of his own ego, or expose himself to the risks and rewards—the dazzle and the glitter—of the infinite universe.

In traditional times, the martial arts master developed his skills and personality in a rarefied environment unencumbered by commercial distractions and tempered by the guiding influence of his teacher. In modern society, the incorporation of the martial arts into one's life does not mean retreating to a secluded cave or monastery, nor disengaging from the pressures and demands of everyday life. Rather, the real enlightenment that is sought after simply means the recognition that serenity and mind-body integration can occur in the context of ordinary life. The person who is patient and focused with regards to the banal and trivial details of everyday existence, will one day have the same patience and focus in mastering the extraordinary and sublime. The martial arts are not about a set of mysteries and secrets accessible only to the most ambitious and talented. Its applications are not limited to the *dojo* or even the street. Everywhere we go and everything we do provides countless opportunities to practice and improve the skills and attitudes we learn as a martial artist. The right means of practice becomes as important as the ultimate objective.

The true martial artist, as perpetual student, is always training at some level to cultivate his *shen* or spirit. Every day, he allocates some time for physical conditioning, technical proficiency or emotional control.

Outsiders who view the martial arts merely as a hobby or a sport might view this type of attitude as fanatical or obsessive. But the martial artist, like the warriors of a bygone age, is seeking exactly the opposite—discipline, balance and control. By pursuing his daily study, he believes that really living fully in his life involves working towards being free of his limitations.

Daily training does not mean relentless exhausting workouts. Proper martial training involves not only physical practice but also academic study and quiet reflection. Work, rest and play is an integral part of effective training. The psychology of training is as important as technique and physical conditioning. In the beginning, the novice may pay too much attention to learning the proper form of a technique without understanding the principle underlying that technique. Until he does, he is merely acting mechanically like a robot. As time passes, he will learn the situational rationale for applying the technique and then become exposed to its variations. While the form may be imperfect, what is more important now is the student's process of observation. He should be aware of what is happening in his body, and in the relative position of his opponent. At this point, the first of many veils may be lifted, as the student begins to understand not just what he does but also why.

Practice and repetition are essential in striving towards proficiency, but only up to a point. To practice a technique ten more times just for quantity's sake is self-defeating if no thought is given to form or to concept. To exercise when the body is overtired does not make one's body adapt better to conditioning. To train when the mind is distracted risks the acquisition of bad habits and brings on the stagnation of mental boredom. When a student practices techniques, he should do them as he would in real life when someone is threatening him. What does that mean exactly? It means that when he throws a punch, launches a kick or makes a block, he acts as if every move he makes counts and has consequences.

How much time and effort should a student practice a move that he will not have the confidence to use in real life? For example, other than for balance and coordination, should he spend much time practicing kicks with the left leg (for most people, this is the weak leg) if he fully intends to use the right leg for fighting? When students in the *dojo* spar, they often try out fancy moves that are in the system or that they have seen in movies such as jumping spinning rear kicks to the head or complex multiple strikes. Since a student typically has a limited amount of time in his life to devote to his art, when he practices, he should "practice real life." Martial arts are a form of personal combat and should be treated as if our life depended on it.

Martial arts techniques are most effective when they are executed with strength, speed and flexibility. Practitioners of more linear styles appreciate the aggressive and direct nature of their techniques, while devotees of circular styles emphasize a redirection of force. Most styles have both a hard physical aspect and a soft subtle aspect. The mature martial artist develops a sensibility to the duality of all things: hard and soft, fast and slow, ferocious and silent. He balances the dichotomy of pacifism and violence, and reconciles the contradictions of solitariness and community.

Many martial arts techniques are designed to inflict serious injury or death. There are lethal techniques in martial arts systems for such specific moves as wrist and elbow breaks, chokes, eye gouges, nerve point striking and leg sweeps. A correctly applied choke can bring about brain damage or death; a strike or kick can maim permanently; techniques applied against nerve or pressure points can cause excruciating pain and unconsciousness. Techniques of attack are designed to exploit the predictable involuntary response of the opponent so that he is vulnerable to a finishing blow. The objective of an effective response is not just to counter or parry a strike; it is to shut down an opponent's ability to function. That is why the study of a martial art must be undertaken seriously and only under a qualified teacher.

Proficiency in techniques is insufficient unless the student is fully committed to executing them. When these techniques were first created centuries ago, they were meant for practitioners who often faced life-threatening situations. Their goal was survival and the vanquishing of an opponent. For example, a defensive move against a knife-wielding attacker was not designed to avoid the knife and restrain the attacker by grabbing his wrist and arm; it was to avoid the knife and simultaneously break his wrist, and then followed by a deadly finishing blow. In that era, training and tournaments were extremely violent, often resulting in injury and death. Understandably, many aspiring martial artists were reluctant to sacrifice their bodies in order to learn the art.

In today's society, there is a more moderate way of training that enables the student to learn techniques with control and without too much physical pain. Instructors take care to limit the full effect of such techniques in order to avoid inflicting pain towards fellow students. Proper training helps the student ascend towards a higher level of control. The biggest challenge facing martial arts students today is that many are not willing or able to make the necessary investment in time, effort and discipline. As a result, they may not be able to develop the mental attitude that facilitates true learning. Even for those who willingly undergo the demanding challenges required of their bodies—the aches and pains, the occasional injury—they may not be prepared to pursue the martial Way as both a development of physical skills and the development of character.

*The good man does not grieve that other people
do not recognize his merits. His only anxiety is lest
he should fail to recognize theirs.*

— Confucius

We are not born into this world for ourselves alone.

— Plato

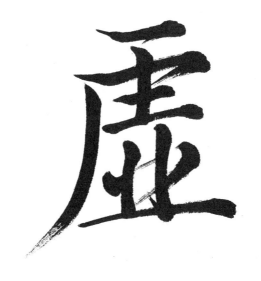

shu (Chn.)
emptiness

Lose Your Ego | VI

The martial arts carry within its practice a paradox. In one respect, it could be viewed as an egotistical, self-absorbed art. When the practitioner goes to the *dojo* to train, for whom is he really doing it for? Is the conditioning of his body and mind done for the benefit of his family and friends? Does learning to become a better fighter in any way advance the interests of his circle of acquaintances? One apparent answer is that he does the martial arts for himself alone. Whether in solitary practice or in group training, only the individual martial artist knows how much real effort he is putting into the art and therefore how much benefit he might derive from it. In truth, although the *sifu* has some responsibility for his student's progress, nobody else honestly cares that much. Yet if one were to ask any serious martial artist, he would say that the martial arts has nothing to do with advancing one's own selfish interests or taking advantage of others. In fact, the ethos of humility, restraint and unselfishness is so ingrained in martial arts culture that anyone who violates these precepts are quickly ostracized by his peers. This apparently contradictory motivation in martial arts training has its roots in the Buddhist and Taoist philosophies that spawned its historical development.

The guiding principal of the Tao is a release of oneself from selfishness. A person reaches this state of enlightenment only by the constant repetition of and adherence to the ideals of the Way, not only in the conscious mind, but also in the heart and soul. True traditional martial arts training cuts through egotism and fear. The practice of the martial arts, as in life, is to strengthen one's physical skills and spirit. When a person tries too hard to lose his ego, he only gets caught up within it. As long as he lives and breathes, he can never rid himself of his ego. However, he can learn to banish its domineering nature and relegate it to the background of his mind. Students of the martial arts aim not only towards the mastery of their chosen art but also towards emptying their minds of materialistic attachments and their hearts of egotistical vanity, literally to forget the self. It is unnecessary to try so hard "to win"; only then can one truly win.

A central tenet in both Taoism and Zen Buddhism is the notion of emptiness. This is well illustrated by the anecdote of a "robber entering an empty house." If a house is empty of all possessions, then a robber has no conceivable motivation for entering the dwelling. Even if he does enter it, finds nothing to take and then leaves, can it be said that he has committed a crime? What is this state in which the motivation for selfish intentions has been removed, and there is nothing valuable to be taken away. The Zen mind would call this serenity or freedom!

Zen philosophy teaches us that our attachment to material things is the root cause of our suffering. When one moves away from the inclination to attach oneself to things, and towards a more detached mind in which all things are observed, then one has entered the realm of emptiness. When a person looks at a tree, he can focus on one leaf and not see the whole tree. If he focuses on every leaf, his mind becomes overwhelmed with detail; but if he concentrates on a leaf, then on the whole tree, then on nothing at all, then he has approached emptiness and has a chance of seeing everything he needs to see. In the martial arts context, when the martial artist is physically relaxed and mentally calm, he is in a controlled state of coordination where the body is synchronized with the mind. Similarly, to truly see others, one must step outside of the circle that constantly presses from without. Don Juan has described this process as "stopping the world" in order to "see" it.[19]

There is a term in Zen nomenclature called *mushin* that translates loosely as the "absence of a conscious mind" (literally "no-mind"), and its Chinese equivalent is roughly *shu*. This concept, while seemingly simple, is one of the most fundamental ideas in Buddhism and also in the martial arts. It refers to a state where the martial artist is not consciously aware of the details of his techniques. The physical act is automatic and free, as if no conscious thought has interfered with it. In this state, the mind moves from one sequence to another, like a stream of water flowing downhill. With sufficient practice and self-confidence, physical movements become instinctive and immediate. One movement follows another without the interruption of the conscious mind. In the martial arts context, Bruce Lee described it this way: "Moving, be like water. Still, be like a mirror. Respond like an echo."[20] Free of judgement and presupposition, the mind is free to act instinctively.

The 1973 film classic *Enter the Dragon* catapulted both Bruce Lee and the martial arts onto the consciousness of the world stage. In the opening scene of the original uncut version, Lee is instructing a young boy how to perform a high kick. At first, the boy kicks in good form but stops just short of the target in a demonstrative pose. Lee immediately chastises him and says: "What is that? Do you think you are in an exhibition? We need emotional content. Try again." The boy kicks again with exertion and a grimace on his face. But Lee scolds him again and says: "I said with emotional content, not anger!" The boy begins to protest and says: "But I thought..." Lee interrupts him and says: "Don't think. Just feel." Finally, the boy launches a kick to his instructor's satisfaction. The kick is in perfect form, with power and fluidity, while the boy's face remains calm and controlled. Alas, the young student was concentrating on his technique, while his teacher was trying to teach him some spiritual insight. In a scientific endeavor, one needs to know the facts; but in an art, the facts are less important. It is a matter of right feeling. Rather than adhering strictly to theory or technique, the martial artist trusts in what feels right.

The reality of day-to-day life is comprised of a continuous flow of perceptual interpretations. A focus on the big picture and being in the present moment helps a person from being inundated with trivial details. As a result, even in the most unexpected moment, one will be ready to cope with danger and adversity. By practicing without egotistical ideas, the martial artist expresses his understanding of the art. When the kicks and strikes of an experienced martial artist is observed, it appears so natural and effortless; but the casual observer cannot even imagine the thousands of hours of diligent training that went into even a short routine. With the mind and body acting in concert, one may contemplate how an opponent might attack and what the response should be. When a student practices this over and over again, the proper response becomes part of his subconscious. When someone is actually attacking, there is no time to think. Strangely enough, in the heat of combat, thinking interferes with fighting. If an individual has no choice but to fight, then he must fight with instinct and strength. It is the time for action, not thinking. Due to the reflex action of the conditioned subconscious, the body can put forth its highest skill. This is the highest point when consciousness becomes one with the body. The repetition of planned responses to stress and external threats contributes to a sense of mastery among martial artists capable of peak performance.

Every form of martial arts employs the use of preset patterns by which a master teaches a student. The traditional practice of *kata* or forms, the prearranged sequence self-defense movements, is a device that not only reinforces knowledge of techniques but also engenders a detached mind. It is passed down from generation to generation in more or less the same way, assimilating centuries of accumulated knowledge. For the uninitiated, the practice of *kata* may seem like mindless repetition. But for those who understand it, *kata* is the very essence of combat training because it perfectly aligns form and application. The martial artist who performs *kata* correctly sees in his mind the exact execution of a technique as he performs it. The repeated fusion of mental imagery and physical application ensures that the martial artist can truly learn to defend himself. He learns a sense of his own bodily rhythm and the center of his own physicality.

In every single technique, there are so many variations, angles and other subtleties involved in its mastery that *kata* is often the best way to learn them. The linking of a mental image with the physical movement programs the mind and the body to respond correctly and spontaneously. When a martial artist performs a *kata* well, it is only because he has spent much time and effort to learn it. An enormous amount of work and thought is involved in perfecting forms so that it appears to the observer as if the performance is done with ease and clarity. The ideal result is the observation of a dazzling performance, pleasurable for both the artist and the audience. Yet it is almost impossible for the performer to be actively "thinking" about the *kata* at the instant he is doing it. In the practice of *kata*, it is the body alone that should be active, while the mind remains passive, watchful and alert. The mind is visualizing rather than participating, so that it can monitor the body's mistakes. The mind becomes a mirror, resembling the smooth surface of a pond, calm and undistracted as the body goes through its rehearsed movements. The physical breathing is steady and uniform, in tandem with the regular pulsation of the heart and the brain. With the proper understanding of what *kata* is, the practitioner realizes that it is principally an exercise for the mind to become fully integrated with the body. More than physical exercise, *kata* closes the loop between the brain and the rest of the body. It is via this process that the real learning of martial arts skills takes place.

The physical exercise of *kata* is a spiritual exercise that is intended to modify and transform the student who practices it. It is a form of internal dialogue or meditation that helps the martial artist progress in his training from within. The mental discipline needed in practicing *kata* is also useful in developing a calm detachment during the heat of combat. Dave Lowry has described a simple device called "viewing the distant mountain" that helps the fighter perceive all the details of a confrontation and yet remain somewhat removed from it.[21] It calls for staring slightly past the shoulder of the opponent without acknowledging any eye contact, as if one were viewing a mountain in the distance. Therefore, one's sight is focused on nothing in particular and yet everything in general, comparable to our metaphor of seeing both the leaves and the tree. Of course, this mental posturing also enables the martial artist to adopt a more transcendent perspective on all other aspects of his training.

There are many ways that one can bend the mind towards a transcendent posture. Self-detachment helps separate consciousness from other undesirable behaviors. Alternatively, direct intervention by self or others whenever a negative pattern of thought or action occurs can help modify the entrenched attitudes and habitual responses in the brain. When there is no desire for the world to be different from what it is, a warrior's mind is free of judgement. Without psychological insecurity or fear, there is no reason to be argumentative or confrontational, no unnecessary battles to fight. This exhilarating sense of freedom and acceptance allows the warrior to act spontaneously and to move through the world without any attention to himself.

In the martial arts, it is futile to use acquired skills to impress others. A contest between two opponents or against others in a tournament is simply a sporting event, nothing more. They carry little lasting value and serve to distract the martial artist from his true mission. The most dangerous traps for the serious martial artist are the emotions and attitudes that might hinder his training and physical well being. These are the feelings of overconfidence, selfishness, and aggressiveness. The martial artist trains to become stronger and physically skilled. He practices fighting with others. He unwittingly also fights with himself. Essentially what he is really doing is figuring how to get beyond winning and losing, success and failure, inner peace and inner conflict. If not, then the martial arts are merely a sport, a game or a business. As such, it contributes little to one's spiritual life and may not hold much enduring value.

The mightiest warrior leaves no trace of destruction.
The swiftest runner leaves no trace of footsteps.
The greatest poet leaves few words.

—Lao Tzu

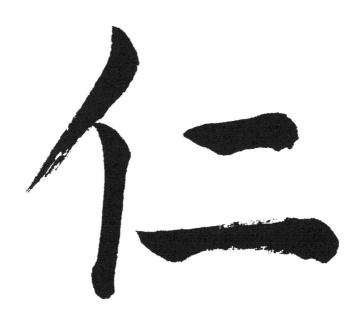

ren
goodness

The Illusion of Technique VII

In the classic *Tao of Jeet Kune Do*, Bruce Lee taught us that the heart of martial arts lies in understanding techniques. The secrets and insights of hundreds of years of martial arts are embedded in the condensed movements of formal techniques. A good technique involves many variations in speed, angle and adaptability. Lee advised the practice of technique until they are a part of oneself, to "put the heart of the technique into your own heart."

Yet in an obvious paradox, the very essence of Lee's philosophy stresses the transcendence of a total reliance upon any system of techniques or forms. A rigid system may lead a practitioner to become a robot repeating routines that are abstract and not fully understood. Instead of responding to a real life situation, he gets ensnared in a pattern of movements and conceptualizations that he has literally practiced to death. A martial arts style that is not open and adaptable may offer a dead end instead of a vehicle for continual learning. Lee advocates that the true martial artist abandons the whole notion of a style, in fact, to go beyond a system. A style that is closed and mechanical also causes the person to think in a way that is closed and mechanical. Responses based on set patterns inevitably become narrow and limiting. In contrast, real life fighting is chaotic, unpredictable and without rules. It requires a response that is immediate and direct. Whether a system emphasizes kicking, striking, grappling, or throwing, they are all part of the underlying fundamentals of any martial arts training. The martial artist employs all the techniques he can to serve his ends. This is the meaning of the often-repeated maxim of "learning techniques in order to go beyond technique".

In a paraphrasing of a well-known concept described by the Zen master Taisen Deshimaru, Lee offered us the following insight:

> Before I studied the art, a punch to me was just a punch, a kick was just a kick. After I'd studied the art, a punch was no longer a punch, a kick was no

longer a kick. Now that I understand the art, a
punch is just a punch, a kick is just a kick.[22]

What does Lee's play on words mean? Metaphorically, it closely resembles the three stages of Zen Buddhists in training. The first stage (termed the *"shiho"* or the *"transmission"*) requires great conscious effort and some five years of diligent practice. As a novice learning the martial arts, he is taught the basic techniques that serve as the building blocks of training. Although he practices them thousands of times faithfully, they are sometimes repeated in a mechanical fashion, without sufficient thought given to subtlety, variability and meaning. At this rudimentary level of training, even though he practices, he improves only slowly and knows that he is not very skillful. Hence, "a punch is just a punch,…"

However, when he becomes more advanced, he has experienced many instances when a given technique fails miserably in real life; or it works in only one circumstance but not in another; or by changing one seemingly trivial detail, the technique becomes transformed into something much more lethal. At this middle level, he is still no real threat to an experienced opponent, but he is aware of his deficiencies, and he recognizes the weaknesses of others. This roughly corresponds to the second stage of Zen training wherein the disciple is on his way towards self-mastery. At this point, he begins to understand how mastery of techniques is a lifelong endeavor that requires both sustained practice and ongoing real life experience. He begins to appreciate the depth of the art and the true challenge of achieving mastery. Hence, "a punch is more than just a punch…"

At the highest levels, the martial artist gains confidence in his own abilities and carefully chooses his own path. He is now a proficient martial artist whose skills are recognized by others and, in turn, respects the skills of others. In most cases, this might be the best that he can aspire to. But on an even higher level, after many years of development and reflection, he finally recognizes the reality that while he may be a good martial artist, the pursuit of perfection is always beyond his grasp. There is no end to training and he may never be completely satisfied with his efforts. At that point, he may adjust both his mind and his body to focus on more limited, attainable goals. He has seen all the strategies and the situations and has become more adaptable. The veteran martial artist treasures the power of simplicity. He simplifies his training to those aspects that he enjoys the most and is the most effective at. He avoids the use of a complex technique when a simple one will do. He returns to basics in order to become more complete instead of simply relying upon raw talent. He knows that the difference between victory and defeat is often the result of paying attention to simple things. Rather than impressing himself or others with his extensive knowledge, what he cares about now are the techniques and the concepts that work well. As a teacher of the martial arts, he rejects obfuscation and mysticism and tries to impart his wisdom in a simple and concrete way. By doing so, he uses the simplest language and draws from the situations of everyday life. Now that he understands the art, he can truly say that "a punch is just a punch, and a kick is just a kick."

The "illusion of technique" is seductive because it implies that if one practices enough the right method and follows the right procedure, then mastery of the martial arts will be the result. A person who imitates techniques in isolation can never become a complete martial artist. There can be no perfection based solely on the refinement of technique. Technique not embedded in some sort of decisive philosophy is just an elaborate form of physical exercise. It is only when each technique, each physical movement is done in coordination with mind and body does real learning take place. The mastery of technique is only one component of training.

Darrell Craig, in his historical analysis of *jujitsu* in *Japan's Ultimate Martial Art*, has argued that the development of a true practitioner must embrace the essential three elements of technique (*waza*), spirit (*shen*) and energy (*ki or chi*). This is really just another way of interpreting the principal of mind-body integration. The physical techniques of the martial arts are part of but can exist independently of the spiritual aspects of the art. We can spend years perfecting the many techniques for hitting and blocking without understanding or digesting any deeper meaning behind the technique. As such, the martial arts become sport and are no different than many other forms of physical activity. In traditional martial arts training, martial spirit evolves from the ongoing practice of technique, and *chi* is a natural result of the development of spirit. The virtue of practicing technique a thousand times, under the proper circumstances, is that it simultaneously enhances all aspects of the martial artist.

Without the proper supervision and guidance of an appropriate teacher, the person who concentrates solely on technique will invariably become discontented and disappointed with his training. Conversely, the essential concepts underlying the martial arts can be intellectually understood, up to a point, without any prolonged physical involvement. Those who care only for the physical aspect of training may become muscular and drenched in sweat, brimming with physical excitement and strength, well anchored in the tangible dimension like rock and earth, but lacking any real appreciation of the art. At the same time, those who are only enamored of the idealism and intellectualization of the martial arts will be blind to the compelling and rough-and-ready reality of real life training. They are like a piece of glass, brittle and fragile when juxtaposed with the blood and sweat of physical exertion. The complete martial artist strives to bring these two worlds together.

Formalized techniques in any style are typically passed over many generations of students. They are not necessarily ends in themselves but just a way of passing down a body of knowledge to posterity. For any given technique, some may work better for certain individuals and in certain contexts, but it is the student's job to understand the essence of the technique before he casually tries to adapt it for his own circumstances. However, an intellectual understanding of technique by itself is empty. The martial arts are not merely about a set of techniques, but about highly developed physical control and spirituality. Through training, the student develops the insight to use the physical tools of his body effectively. No matter how good techniques are, they are only as good as the mental acuity and spiritual insight one draws upon to utilize them. That is how the martial artist uses his skills and knowledge to face whatever confronts him.

Tri Thong Dang, in his meditation on the art of discipleship *Beyond the Known*, has described the ultimate goal of the martial arts this way:

> *When he reached that state in which technique is not considered, only then could he emanate from the center of his being, that place where body and mind and spirit dance as one. Only then when intellect was no longer conscious, when body was no longer monitored, when spirit was no longer engaged, was he embodying the artless art.*[23]

Learning a new technique without truly understanding or assimilating those that have already been taught is counterproductive in two respects. First, it gives a false perception of learning new material where no such process may have yet occurred. Second, it generates additional clutter from which the mind/body must extricate itself if it is to digest the original data that is already in process. The capacity to improvise techniques in a spontaneous way is severely limited unless the martial artist has a strong grounding in the basics of his original style.

Many students who train in traditional styles have multiple objectives for their training. Often the ability to fight effectively for self-defense is an important by-product of learning the art though it may not have been the original primary motivation. A student who learns the art under an experienced instructor knows that only a small minority of the techniques that are taught will ever be actually used for personal combat. However, he learns all of the techniques in a given system so that he has multiple tools in his repertoire of skills to draw upon and enjoy through the course of his life. By gaining insight into his own strengths and weaknesses, he learns firsthand the qualities of humility and perseverance so essential to mastering any martial arts style. At the higher levels, the emergence of the martial spirit, in conjunction with a heightened awareness, enables the practitioner to use *chi* and subtlety of technique in place of mere muscle for effective self-defense.

To perfect a technique is to face the paradox of knowing that such technical perfection is virtually unattainable. The martial artist falls short because of the limitations of his own ability and the random circumstances of real-life physical confrontations. Techniques that work for one student may be inappropriate for another. The student can only work towards finishing and understanding the task before him. In time, the satisfaction of accomplishment will be achieved through practice. Consequently, it is important to preserve as much as possible martial systems in their entirety for the benefit of posterity. When teachers learn and pass on the insights and skills embedded in a system, they honor the cumulative wisdom and accomplishments of past martial arts masters.

Since mastery is more of an ideal than an actuality, humility is always more appropriate than self-satisfaction. A student learns techniques from his teacher but, at some point, he needs to surpass what he has been taught. He must begin to create for himself, to go "beyond the known." Imitation lacks spirituality, and implies an absence of originality. At the highest levels, conventional techniques are transcended. Isn't that why the martial arts is called an "art"?

Do not move unless it is advantageous.
Do not execute unless it is effective
Do not challenge unless it is critical.
                                    —*Sun Tzu*

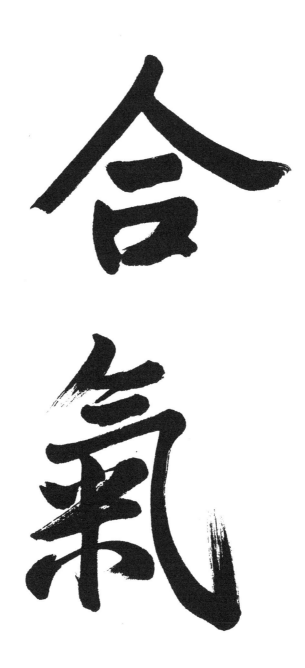

aiki (Jap.)
harmony of mind and body,
leading to an impassive state of mind

Circles and Straight Lines | VIII

In the heat of battle, the warrior must determine what is the best way to deal with force. If such force cannot be avoided, then it is better to redirect it. Since the martial artist believes that life is precious, he finds more ways to preserve rather than to destroy. Classical warriors, battlefield strategists, and martial arts masters all know that there are just three ways to respond to an enemy's attack. The first is avoidance, retreating and positioning oneself out of harm's way. This is usually advisable when one is not fully prepared or when the opponent enjoys overwhelming strength. The second response is evasion, avoiding the enemy's initial attacks while staying within close range, hoping to find the opportune moment to retaliate. Evasion is risky and requires extensive experience and finesse. Finally, the third response is interception, an aggressive, direct counterattack against the opponent in hopes of a quick victory. Obviously, interception is advisable only when one is confident that available resources and tactics are stronger than the other side. When one is faced with a vulnerable and weaker opponent, sometimes the most straightforward response is to intercept his advance with crushing force.

The above strategy applies to all circumstances of personal defense as well as to martial arts tactics. Many martial arts styles such as *judo* and *karate* rely on a straight-line concept of leverage in their techniques. Force at one end of a lever must be countered with another force across the fulcrum. In many instances, a straight line to the objective is both the simplest and the most effective response. A direct, linear attack avoids all unnecessary gestures. The fighter is single-minded as he advances forward upon his quarry. But unless the fighter can also control the speed of his advance and adjust for the distance between oneself and the target, the strike may come too late and miss its target. Having a sense of time is to become aware of the space in which motion takes place.

In contrast, *aikido* (arguably the most explicitly spiritual of the modern martial arts styles) emulates the balance wheel of a circular watch wherein force is controlled by balancing motion with mass. The *karate* stylist learns to break hard objects with his bare hands by utilizing a mental technique in which he aims for the far side of the target object. He projects his force in a straight line through the object. *Aikido* relies heavily on the same concept of projection but in a circular motion. Unlike straight-line motion that can only be regulated with brute force, circular motion is easier to control and direct. Circles can be narrowed as in a spiral, or widened as it opens into a straight line.

The underlying philosophy of circular motion is that the "life force" (*chi* in Chinese or *ki* in Japanese) circulates in a dynamic circle that never closes or ends. This dynamic sphere moves toward infinity; and the ever-changing circle can be as small as the circumference of a single point or as large as a fraction of an arc on an infinite circle. It redefines human confrontation by turning defensive resistance into an advantage. This orientation draws from the Chinese strategic board game of *weichi* (or Japanese *go*) that builds on the perception of controlling an adversary by encircling him.

Who would want to face an angry opponent rushing head-on into a fight? (Figure 1) In most instances, it is better to evade the thrust of a direct attack than to face it head on. The concept of yielding in the face of force is one of the most fundamental ideas in the martial Way. If an opponent is much bigger and stronger, it is better to find a way not to fight. Why risk bodily harm unnecessarily? On the other hand, if one is bigger and stronger than the opponent, it is possible to take advantage of such a direct confrontation. In real life, this scenario is unlikely since smaller, weaker people typically do not directly attack larger, stronger ones. In either case, although even if a person may have stopped an attack momentarily, he has not positioned himself for the inevitable subsequent moves of his adversary (Figure 2).

The fundamental premise of *aikido* is to redirect the opponent's strength away from oneself and never to directly confront that strength. Circling away from an oncoming force, changing its direction, pushing it from behind, and rendering it harmless is the essence of *aikido*. In this way, the principal of circles and straight lines is analogous to water and stone. A stone is hard and immovable, until it is shattered by an even greater force, or is swept away by the flowing water, or is eventually eroded by the effects of water and wind. But like the skilled martial artist, water yields without hesitation, and slips away elusively from the opponent's clutches. This concept of yielding is central to *aikido* and to many other martial arts styles as well. To be flexible and "loose" implies greater coordination, agility and smoothness of motion. In physical terms, it refers to the controlled relaxation of the limbs, joints, muscles and tendons of the body. Only in this state can power be economically transmit-

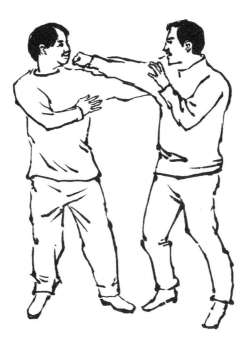

Figure 1. Linear Attack Finds Its Target.

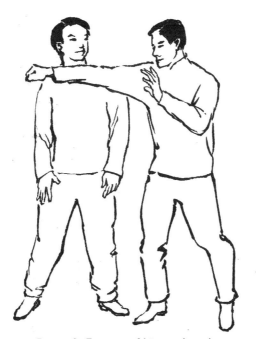

Figure 2. Evasion of Linear Attack.

ted from its conception to the target.

Since the true martial artist rarely initiates a violent attack, most offensive actions are responses to or an anticipation of a threatening movement. It involves physical maneuvering, evasion and a plan of counter-attack. The process of attack is psychophysical, encompassing the brain, muscles and nerves. The mental assessment of the situation then dictates the crucial variables of timing, distance, angle and power. The intelligent fighter is both mentally and physically alert, and he will change his tactics in response to the actions of his opponent and the particulars of the situation. This means that he must closely observe the strengths and weaknesses of his opponent. For example, a circular offensive movement may not be effective if the other person responds with a straight parry or counter-attack. Likewise, a direct punch without any feints is unlikely to reach the opponent who adeptly moves off the centerline in a circular evasion. Therefore, tactics are always predicated on the opponent's reactions and habits.

Even though the martial artist may be engaged in combat, his mind and his behavior should not be too different from his everyday manner. He should appear as if nothing critical is happening. His movements, whether linear or circular, have a clear function. Any combative situation can be charted in two or more circles. When the opponent has penetrated the circle of the target, he must respond. But until that point, he should maintain his distance and control, moving in concentric circles where the innermost circle represents his sphere of control. When an opponent is pulled into the target's own circle or enters it voluntarily to initiate an attack, he creates an opening in his own circle of defense. That is the time to counterattack. One moves just enough to evade the attack, and redirects the path of the opponent's energy back against him or in a straight line that causes him to lose his balance. In geometric terms, the arc of the opponent's curve meets one's own circle and gets redirected into a spiral or a tangent. The attacker's motion can thus be redirected anywhere at will (Figures 3 & 4).

Evasion from attack is actually quite an aggressive art. Fading, ducking and slipping are all tactics that are used for protection while positioning oneself for a counterattack. Attack by deception involves both evasion and feinting. Feinting requires using the body and eyes to fool the opponent, and to make him reveal his plan. An unexpected hand movement, a shuffling of the feet or a sudden yell can distract the opponent and make him lose concentration. When an opponent is confused or trying to adjust his moves to a perceived feint, it creates a momentary opening that can be exploited. The winning fighter knows how to use this temporary opening to launch his own attack.

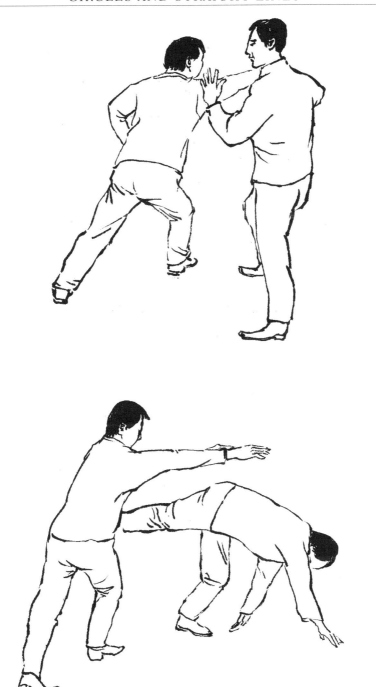

Figures 3 & 4. Evasion and Redirection of Attack via Outward Circular Motion.

The decision to decisively enter an opponent's inner circle of space requires both courage and self-confidence. It is undoubtedly safer to deal with an adversary from a distance, but in order to effect a throw or land a blow, one must enter into the opponent's center and control it. If a fighter only tries to conserve energy and avoid the blows of his opponent, he cannot win. An inability to do this renders a fighter totally ineffective. To successfully counter, the fighter must evade the strike and land his own strike while the opponent is out of position as a result of our evasive movement. Sometimes a quick direct strike will shock the opponent, especially when he is expecting something much more elaborate. The element of surprise can compensate for the opponent's superiority in size, strength or technical skill. The counterattack, like the evasive movement, also demands a high skill level. It is not so much a defensive response as it is a means of using the opponent's offensive techniques to create a line of attack. Consequently, it demands a mastery of technique, mental calculation, timing and control. Keep the opponent on the defensive, do not let him regroup, concentrate on his weaknesses, and always keep him guessing (Figures 5 & 6).

The capacity to out-maneuver and out-think our opponent is required for success in total fighting. Through long practice, martial artists learn to deliver the right combination of punches and kicks at the right strength, and at the right time. With proper training, the body does this spontaneously, freeing the mind to respond at will to an opponent's moves. The tactics a fighter chooses to use is the essence of fighting. By analyzing the opponent's strengths and weaknesses, he then constructs his own plan. Then the proper execution of the attack must be applied quickly and without hesitation. Through practice, the controlled reaction of muscles and limbs become automatic, and the brain can concentrate on the strategy and tactics needed to win the fight. During the time of actual fighting, there is not enough time to think carefully because one must act. But the outcome of the fight is dependent on the brain, not the hands and feet. Mechanical control, the coordination of mind and body, and an intelligent analysis of the opponent all come together in a champion.

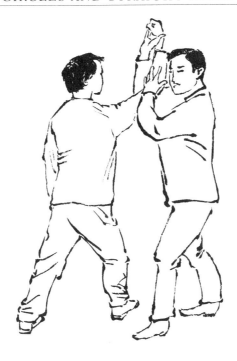

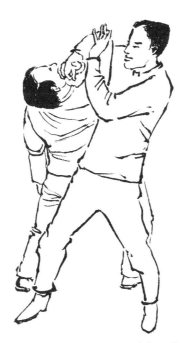

Figures 5 & 6. Deflection and Redirection of Attack via Inward Circular
Motion.

PART III

Water will seek its own level.
It is the nature of water to do so.
Unrestricted by the opinions of rocks in the stream,
it goes where it will and is patient to do so.
                              —*Lao Tzu*

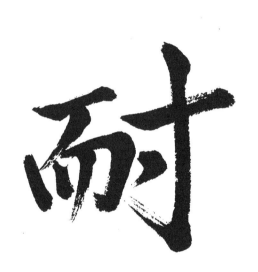

nai
patience

Time and Timing | IX

An individual does not merely exist in space but is defined by his physical place in this world. Similarly, he does not merely exist in time but is affected by the passage of time. The consciousness of time dominates a person's life, particularly as he ages. It is time that gives him a sense of past and future and impels him through his days. The experience of whether time passes quickly or slowly is often determined by how an individual reacts to common events as well as unexplored emotions. In the martial arts, learning and achieving involves both the process and the product. The profound influence of Buddhism on the development of the martial arts is critical in helping the student understand the role of time in his training.

A well-known aphorism from the classic Buddhist texts illustrates the larger Buddhist conception of human life and time: "The elephant is the wisest of all the animals, the only one who remembers his former lives, and he remains motionless for long periods, meditating thereon." Like the allegorical elephant in question, the martial artist's focus is always on "the present moment" and then subsequently on "a lifetime" of training. Thus he is relieved of the absurd emphasis on the short term, the pressure for instant gratification, and the stupefying ten-step formulaic approach to achievement. When he approaches a task without an arbitrary time limit, he can then focus on the work without the attendant anxiety. By understanding the value of practice, he can approach his training easily because he can see the wished for result in his mind. Then he simply proceeds to do his work and allows the results to emerge in their own due time.

In life there is a constant need to balance and readjust the mind to the demands of the past, present and future. The true warrior ponders the future without discarding the past while living in the present. The temporal process both separates and unifies a person's perceived experience. The future not only imposes hopes and goals but also deadlines, possible disappointments and the threat of failure. The past is replete with both fond memories and bitter regrets. In between the two, one is left only to face the present. Just as an individual can die at any time, he is also embedded in the moment-to-moment passing of time. The experience of time, and what one can recover from it, is up to each individual. This freedom is affirmative and descriptive of the martial artist in total alertness and openness. By fully engaging in the present moment, he does not dissipate his physical, mental and emotional energies, neither on events that have not yet transpired nor on past events that he is powerless to change. For example, it is futile to compare oneself with a younger, stronger or more skilled opponent and wish that one were younger or stronger. Every martial artist must recognize his own limitations and try to narrow the gap by other means.

Sun Tzu, in his classic 300 B.C. text *The Art of War*, advised that it is best to win without fighting, and if necessary, to fight once rather than twice. The strategist picks his time and place, when the circumstances are most favorable, and then moves quickly. His posture is always to use one's strengths and exploit the opponent's weaknesses. His attitude is always pragmatic: "Avoid losses by avoiding battles you cannot win and fight no battles you are not sure of winning."

Periodic silence and pauses are an integral part of martial arts sparring. Attack and defense do not always occur relentlessly. In attacking, it is useful to pause and observe the reactions of the opponent before continuing. This not only allows us to reassess the effectiveness of our strategy but also serves to confuse the opponent as to the next move. A traditional Japanese saying advises us that fish do not live in clear water. In order for fish to be able to evade its predators and grow to maturity, it must be able to hide behind the seaweed and to lose itself in the rocks and sand. Thus, it is the same way in human confrontations. In the midst of sparring, a variety of attacks and defenses tend to confuse the adversary, and it also eases the strain of exclusively using one part of the body for the fight. Moreover, it is inadvisable to use the same techniques against every opponent. A good fighter varies his approach and style according to the situation. A martial artist who is well grounded in the techniques of his system can draw upon a wealth of tools to address any situation he faces.

In the face of confrontation, knowing when to retreat and when to stop is crucial in evading a direct collision of brute force. An economy of motion suggests an avoidance of superfluous, extravagant or extreme movements. The experienced martial artist does just what is necessary for self-defense, without over-committing himself by extreme swings or lunges. Instead, he is patient, bides his time and waits for his opponent to overreach before he counterattacks. As he maintains his balance and keeps his block up, he tries to detect when his adversary is at a point of imbalance.

A successful attack also implies a powerful attack. A relaxed movement combined with explosive speed creates a powerful thrust. A tense position results in short, jerky movements. In throwing a punch, the more relaxed the arms, fists and shoulders, the faster and more powerful the punch will become. Relaxation is the prerequisite for precision and power. This means being ready but not tense, being flexible and aware, quietly waiting for whatever may come, and revolving slowly like a wheel in motion.

The concept of timing in fighting is a crucial one, with both a physical and psychological dimension. When two opponents are of roughly equal skill levels, they will circle each other in a sequence of attack, defense and counterattack. The timing of each person's move is prompted by the response of the other, creating a rhythm to the sparring. When the initial rhythm is established, there is a strong tendency on the part of both fighters to continue in this pattern until something disrupts it. The fighter who breaks the rhythm, by making an unexpected movement or through a feigned hesitation via a circular or semi-circular movement, can seize a momentary advantage. This is because the opponent has been lulled for a split second into following through with the previous sequence of movements. Hence, the attacker is creating an opening for his line of attack. However, any slight advantage in initiating an attack or breaking a rhythm must be followed by deliverance of a blow with sufficient speed.

The time to make a move is always when the opponent has already started his movement. By starting one's own move when the opponent is halfway through his, it is easier to catch the opponent off balance both physically and mentally. Thus when the opponent is advancing and about to proceed with his attack, the fighter can first lull him into a trap by reacting as the opponent would expect, or confusing him by apparent disengagement and then launching a counter-attack. At that second, the opponent's body and mind is more preoccupied with attack than defense. This is the way to use timing as an advantage during the brief interval before an opponent can react to one's own plan. This element of surprise lets the fighter choose the precise physical and psychological instant to attack when the opponent is at his weakest. If the martial artist trains habitually with the attitude that, when it really counts, he will have just one chance, then he can concentrate absolutely on that moment in question and apply himself with flawless execution.

Marking the distance between oneself and the opponent is the other crucial factor in winning the fight. The maintenance of a correct fighting distance is a constantly changing variable dependent upon the speed and ability of both combatants. The closing and opening of distance shifts rapidly as each person tries to increase his chances of landing a hit by exploiting an opening and then, in turn, decreases the chances of being hit by retreating to a safe distance. Each individual must learn his own fighting distance so that he can consistently stay out of reach of his opponent, while nevertheless being able to reach that opponent with just a short advance.

Attacks, defensive evasions and counterattacks are only effective if they are executed at the right time and at the right speed. They also require the right attitude. The martial artist confronts the situation and believes that he can win. Although he may feel tension and anxiety, he is mentally prepared for a violent exchange. When his emotional control is conditioned for fear and pain, he can retain his hard-earned skills even during the critical moments of a fight. The martial artist who believes that he will win, who is determined to win, can usually draw upon a reservoir of energy and willpower not available to someone without the proper attitude. This only becomes possible when the martial artist truly believes in the ideals and objectives of his art. As a result, his mental state of mind enables him to perform at his peak capacity when the circumstances require it. Bruce Lee describes the champion very simply: "The real competitor is the one who gives all he has, all the time."

He who learns but does not think, is lost.
He who thinks but does not learn is in great danger.
                                    —Confucius

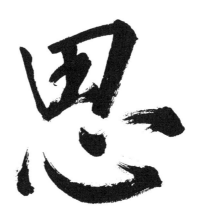

se
thinking

Empower Your Warrior Mind | X

The experienced martial artist is privileged to have undergone a certain kind of training. If he takes his art seriously, he is aware that he carries in his hands the power of life and death. Consequently, he has the responsibility to behave with greater calm and judgement than the average person. The awareness of this responsibility is assimilated into his demeanor. The responsible martial artist does not respond to emotional provocation, because what might typically start out as a mere punch or a shove could easily escalate into something far more serious. The rule of reason, not wounded pride, must govern. The average person responds to the threat of physical assault with fear. Panic can cloud his thinking, perhaps even provoking an extreme self-defense reaction. The martial artist is no stranger to fear, but knows how to manage it. Because of his physical and mental conditioning, he can use all of his mental powers to deflect or escape a violent confrontation. Paradoxically, it is this very attitude and physical bearing that discourages potential attackers. It is axiomatic that the individuals who are most prepared to face deadly force are the ones least likely to have to resort to it. In avoiding potentially lethal conflict, the martial artist becomes the calmest, most moral man on earth.

For example, in the United States there is a very well organized anti-gun lobby that has created a perception that gun owners are often fanatical, paranoid and reckless people who like to carry firearms in order to feed their egos and their aggressiveness. However, if one were to venture into a typical shooting range or gun club, the pervasive mood in such a place is calm and controlled. Law-abiding owners of licensed handguns are all too aware of the power of their weapons. They know that even a seemingly harmless oversight on their part may lead to a deadly tragedy. They also expect the same level of care from other legitimate gun owners. Consequently, there is an inviolate form of etiquette (very similar to that followed by martial artists in the *dojo*) that must be followed when guns are handled on the range or in the presence of other people. All guns must be properly holstered. If they are carried in hand, the well of a revolver or the chamber of an automatic must be open and in clear sight. Guns are always passed to another person with the muzzle pointed away, fingers away from the trigger, and in a slow, deliberate manner. On the range, there are no quick, jerky unexpected physical movements. There is no screaming or raucous laughter. Usually, there is intense concentration, focused practice, and occasional hushed conversation. Like warriors and martial artists, ordinary people who are accustomed to the immediate proximity of lethal weapons respect their awesome power, and therefore act accordingly.

In the development of personal power, a martial artist relies upon a "warrior mind" to provide him with the psychological stability that he needs, to remove the self-doubts and distractions from his mind. When he has attained this self-confidence, his mental focus and spiritual discipline actually enhances his otherwise limited physical strength. In martial arts practice, a strong mental discipline not only intensifies physical strength, it also accelerates achieving mastery of the art. The martial artist has both confidence in his self and faith in his art. This mental resoluteness, and the absence of emotional agitation, is required for the efficient application of techniques. Efficient and decisive responses to attacks allow the fighter to conserve energy and maintain agility. The martial artist's goal is to retain his physical and mental balance while disrupting his opponent's equilibrium. This allows him to deliver his strikes with maximum power. If an opponent makes us enraged, agitated or emotionally unbalanced, he has already gained an advantage. Instead of controlling the situation, the fighter has allowed the opponent to turn the tables against him.

By losing composure, a martial artist reveals his inner feelings to the enemy. Anger at an opponent is a petty indulgence that carries a very high price. Controlling the opponent invariably starts with controlling oneself. A calm, impassive persona keeps the other side off-balanced, unsure of the next move. The ability to hide terror and anger from an adversary is more important than sheer courage and skill. It plants the seed of doubt in an opponent's mind about his own abilities. By redirecting one's negative emotions away from the surface, it can be channeled back, at an opportune moment, like a hidden weapon unleashed in ferocious assault. If the opponent is himself angry, the fighter can exacerbate his adversary's emotional imbalance by provoking him even more. Then the opponent's body will become nervous and tense, and his mind will become encumbered with negative emotions.

The proper martial attitude is, by necessity, a positive attitude. When a martial artist is free from unprovoked threat, he relishes calm and peace. But when he must fight, he must make the transition from self-defense to aggressive offense. The effective fighter always keeps his head up, looking for opportunities, and pushing his abilities. He finds out what his strengths are, and then actually uses them. For example, during sparring a fighter may be reluctant to charge aggressively into an opponent, preferring to stand back to find an opening. Instead of fighting in close and trading blows, he may be more comfortable darting in and out. It is important to recognize one's own style and temperament, to turn what others may view as a weakness into an unanticipated advantage.

In many instances in life, an individual is not defeated by his foes but by himself. Specifically, it is the mental blinders he puts on that limit how he perceives and reacts to adversity. He must face down his own fears and insecurities alone. He has to work through his own physical and mental fatigue without relief from others. If a martial artist trains with narrow expectations, then his ability to call forth his skills and resources is diffident and defeatist. The effectiveness of *karate, judo,* boxing, wrestling and all the rest depends upon the cultivation of mental strength. The body is just a tool for the trained mind. Since the body can only follow the mind, the martial artist develops in tandem his brain, nervous system and muscles so that they can be most efficiently used together. This integration of the ego and the body is sometimes expressed as the development and extension of our life energy or *chi.* When we train regularly and live in an honorable manner, our *chi* flows well and is replenished.

Thinking before acting is the credo of the experienced martial artist. The mind is the most powerful weapon that he possesses. Whether something is difficult or easy is often simply a frame of mind. His arms, legs, elbows and knees are all dependent upon and subservient to the strengths or weaknesses within his head. The application of the mind, as expressed in concepts and words, often has a greater effect on an opponent than wielding a bludgeon. Winston Churchill, arguably the greatest public orator of the twentieth century, knew best how to use words as a weapon. In 1940, when Churchill was asked to lead the British government during England's greatest crisis, he addressed the House of Commons knowing that many of his defeatist colleagues had already lost the will to fight and ready to surrender to the Nazis. With the effect of launching a missile at his enemy, this is what he said:

> *We shall not flag or fail. We shall go on to the end.*
> *We shall fight in France, we shall fight on the seas*
> *and oceans...we shall defend our island, whatever*
> *the costs may be, we shall fight on the beaches, we*

*shall fight on the landing grounds, we shall fight in
the fields and in the streets, we shall fight in the
hills; we shall never surrender.*

It may be too much to analogize the impending defeat of a nation to
the prospect of a personal defeat. Nevertheless, in the face of even the
greatest mortal danger or personal crisis, the mind can remain detached
and choose a rational course. Whatever the situation, a person can react
to the circumstances and not to his anxieties, fantasies and fears. In a life-
threatening situation, it is not simply a matter of physical ability but the
quality of one's mental state. A psychological awareness of the opponent
and the circumstances of the situation may tip the scales in one's favor.
If one were to make no distinctions between victory and defeat, then in
this way one trains the mind to become unbeatable. A true martial artist
will not let himself be defeated because of a narrow mind or a poor attitude.

As the body ages and physical frailties accrue, the fighter must compensate for the failings of his body through greater reliance on experience and wisdom. In this way, pure strength evolves into finesse, and
pure speed evolves into timing. The martial arts are a matter of life and
death. In critical situations the practitioner learns to protect himself as
well as his loved ones. The use of the mind as a weapon comes with time
and experience. If a young person desires to develop these traits in his
youth, he is destined for great things later on in his life. He strives harder, and with more intelligence. Martial arts discipline becomes a life discipline. It is this application of intelligence, fortified by knowledge and
tempered by the wisdom of experience, that makes a martial artist's training complete. The martial artist who practices his craft comes to see that
his techniques are just an extension of his spirit; that his physical world
is part of his spiritual universe. Then he knows that his art, his body, and
his mind are one.

At fifteen, I set my heart upon learning. At thirty, I planted my feet upon the ground. At forty, I no longer suffered from perplexities. At fifty, I knew what were the biddings of Heaven. At sixty, I heard them with docile ear. At seventy, I could follow the dictates of my own heart; for what I desired no longer overstepped the boundaries of right.

— Confucius

He not busy being born is busy dying.

— Bob Dylan

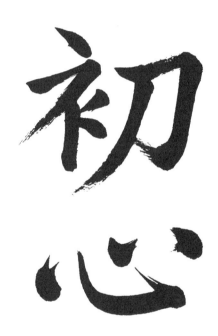

sho shin (Jap.)
beginner's mind

Learning and Teaching | XI

In attaining martial arts knowledge, there are masters and there are disciples. However, the true knowledge that affects the way one lives and dies is not transmitted from teacher to student; it is acquired only by means of personal experience and the performance of concrete acts. As time passes, the ultimate quality of a martial artist hinges more on his state of mind than on his physical ability. Just being able to intellectually understand the martial arts is not enough. What the martial artist learns must be personally experienced and incorporated into his mental, emotional, and physical world.

The aspiring martial artist may use the process of training to realize his own "Zen mind." This just refers to one of those enigmatic phrases that encourages a person to go beyond mere words and to understand his true nature, to go beyond borrowed concepts, to be directly in possession of his own mind, wherever he may be. In the many examples of Zen folklore, the typical practitioner devotes years to emptying his mind; one day, through fatigue and discouragement, his mind finally gives up, empties, and then suddenly intuition and enlightenment occurs spontaneously. The process of self-understanding goes beyond simply gaining knowledge and gathering information. Paradoxically, the attainment of Zen mind is only possible by adopting a "beginner's mind." A beginner's mind is free, empty of preconceptions and bad habits, and ready for all possibilities.

Don Juan, a Native American shaman who certainly never stepped foot inside a Buddhist monastery, has nevertheless described this state of mind in his own inimitable way:

> *We only have two alternatives; we either take everything for sure and real, or we don't. If we follow the first, we end up bored to death with ourselves and with the world. If we follow the second and erase personal history, we create a fog around us, a very exciting and mysterious state in which nobody knows where the rabbit will pop out, not even ourselves.*[24]

The traditional role of master and disciple, and the process of learning and teaching, are well established in Asian cultures. It is particularly crucial for the martial arts practitioner where this form of highly personalized apprenticeship was the rule for nearly two thousand years. To learn the art from a master or any worthwhile teacher is not a simple matter, for it requires a form of physical and mental conversion to the art in question. Unfortunately, this kind of long traditional discipleship is quickly becoming obsolete in modern times. Our society's emphasis on independence, individuality and competition has undermined the perceived importance of undergoing such a sustained and difficult type of training. Moreover, the urge for instant gratification associated with the pursuit of money, power and fame has threatened to reduce the martial arts into a pastiche of fancy techniques, glittery gimmicks, arrogant pseudo-masters, and self-promotional tournaments. Since the business of martial arts has no uniform standards and dubious certification practices, there will occasionally be unscrupulous individuals who will try to convince an audience of a presumed expertise or to promote a new martial arts style. In a world increasingly dominated by celebrity and salesmanship, those who devote themselves to the true virtuous path are, for the most part, unknown and unheard.

The most devoted and effective martial arts teachers are rarely public figures. They merely do what is right for their students and themselves, without fanfare and without casualties. In their work, they embody the virtues of training, moderation and attention to detail. They apply a careful, thoughtful and practical approach to the challenges of everyday life. As a cumulative result, their quiet and inconspicuous example inspires their students and changes the world.

A true martial arts master is someone who continuously practices his art with devotion and passion; and he tries to impart these virtues to his students. The *sifu* or *sensei* is not a salesman or an army drill-sergeant; he does not seek out new students like a stockbroker cold-calling for new clients, nor does he prevent students from leaving his charge. The instructor's role, in the beginning, is to act as a guide as the student embarks on the journey through the martial arts. No matter how skilled he is in his craft, his role is not to impress the student or force his own intentions on him. His responsibility is to help the student master what is within that student's capabilities, while encouraging the student to expand his abilities. A wise teacher does more than simply instruct; he shows the student how to see the things that they still have to learn. The successful teacher helps his students become better martial artists, and not just credible clones of himself. Most importantly, a teacher must embody the principles that he is purportedly teaching. If he tells students it is important to be humble but brags himself, he is both a poor role model and a fool. If he talks about maintaining a calm mind but is himself full of anger, resentment, stress and envy, then his students will quickly hear his heart and not his words.

These days, a search for a good teacher can be a difficult and protracted one. Just as a good teacher is hard to find, being a good student also requires work and commitment. Kensho Furuya once said: "When the student is ready, the teacher will appear."[25] What he meant was that no matter how much a good teacher tries to impart his knowledge to a student, it is useless unless the student is ready to accept such wisdom. However, if a student is sufficiently mature and committed to learning the martial arts, even if a suitable teacher is not immediately nearby, that student through his devotion to the art will eventually find a teacher worthy of his efforts. In the Zen tradition, not only does the master not tell his disciple the answers, he insists that his disciple ask the right questions. In fact, the master instructs his students that if they want to acquire his wisdom, they must "steal" his knowledge. This underscores the idea that true knowledge must be actively acquired, not merely passively received. The gifted teacher helps the student perform in the way that he wants and lets him develop the tools to do it. Such a teacher does not tell the student what to do; he only seems to be pulling the student's thoughts together, to put the student in tune with himself.

If a teacher tells the student to do something, the student should do it until he understands his instructor's intention. If the student does not feel that his teacher is teaching him properly or is not meeting his expectations, then the student should seek another teacher. Whether the student diligently follows the instructor's lead, finds a separate path, or even one day surpasses his teacher, is completely up to the student. But one day if the student feels that he can continue the learning process without close supervision, then he must proceed with the utmost care; for without a guide, even the most advanced student can easily lose his way. Remember that even martial arts masters have masters!

The universal objective for all beginners is to achieve a black belt rank, but few people understand what it is that they want from this. In most cases, the motivation for this desire has more to do with an external confirmation of achievement than for any actual accomplishment. Other distracting motivations are to attain more money, fame, a sense of superiority, control over others, or other selfish goals. When the student understands that the process of training for a black belt is more important than the black belt itself, then he may have a realistic chance of truly earning such a status. The achievement of a first-degree black belt or a *shodan* is not the end of a process but literally the beginning. A *shodan* is a serious student who has demonstrated his ability to learn. He has demonstrated a certain level of physical expertise, and in the conventional sense, has become a formidable fighter. He knows that a lifetime of further training and learning lies ahead, that he is never "good enough," and that the ideals of a true black belt are hard to live by.

At a crucial turning point during World War II, when the Allies defeated the German forces in the summer of 1942 at the Battle of El-Alamein in North Africa, Winston Churchill tried to rally his wounded and exhausted nation against the odious aggression of Nazi Germany. Cognizant of the many battles and dark nights ahead, he said this: " This may not be the end, or even the beginning of the end, but it might be the end of the beginning." So it is for the newly minted black belt! If he feels that he has reached his goal, then he is at the beginning of the end. On the other hand, if he feels that he has just begun his pursuit of self-perfection, then his coveted black belt truly signifies merely the "end of the beginning." Only now does the road to mastery appear before his eyes, beckoning him to continue. The will to persevere in the face of sustained obstacles, and the recognition that a noble goal always requires a high price might also describe the martial artist at a crucial turning point in his maturation.

As the *shodan* continues his training and development, he needs to reinforce his skills and reassess his weaknesses. As he begins to teach other students, he discovers that he learns as much by teaching as when he himself was just a student. Since other junior martial artists now look to him for guidance, a new sense of responsibility emerges. Different systems of martial arts follow varying criteria and requirements for ranking. However, the increasing degrees of black belt rankings do not just correlate to superior levels of fighting ability as measured by speed, power and form. They also reflect the black belt's maturation as an instructor, model and as an individual. At the higher levels (i. e. fifth-degree black belt and above), the concept of martial arts mastery starts to become evident.

Not only does the veteran martial artist now display a seemingly effortless knowledge of principles and techniques, he can apply them to a wide variety of students and circumstances. At the highest levels, physical mastery and mental mastery have become embodied in the same person. To attain this level, the martial artist has served and sacrificed for the sake of his art for decades, well after he has initially achieved his *shodan* rank. Yet, till the day he dies, he must overcome the inclination to be boastful, arrogant, egotistical and competitive. That is the cross that a true black belt must carry. That is why the vast majority of martial arts students never achieve a black belt ranking, and why many black belt holders are not true martial artists. In the end, the martial artist understands that perfecting his true self has nothing to do with rank. Those who seek only the rank and not the substantive content of advancement betray both the spirit and ethos of their chosen art.

The true martial artist is always a student. He is always in the ongoing process of evolving and improving. If he begins to engage in self-promotion or boastfulness, then others may see him not as a master but as a vainglorious fool. If he believes that he has reached the ultimate in his technique, there can be no further growth. The result will be that he will suffer mental stagnation, and other martial artists will feel the same in his presence. The irony is that the aspiring martial artist cannot simply act like a sage or try to emulate one; the mere conscious intention of it nullifies the result. Once again, Confucius says it best: "He who from day to day is conscious of what he still lacks, and from month to month never forgets what he has already learnt, may indeed be called a true lover of learning."

Instead, if the dedicated martial artist never becomes complacent about his present understanding, then he is capable of performing familiar routines in a completely new way. The warrior keeps his swords immaculate; the businessman keeps his desk clear; the painter cleans his brushes; and the martial artist helps to keep his *dojo* clean. The pursuit of perfection is not simply the result of ongoing training; perfection lies within the training itself. The wise teacher understands that his students are merely vehicles for his own ongoing learning. The teacher progresses because teaching is itself a form of learning. Even the triumphant warrior knows that he still needs an attendant to care for his equipment, a mentor to motivate him, a lover to rejuvenate his heart, and loyal retainers to give him a sense of purpose. Finally, the sage understands that training is not an external concept that leads to a goal, but is intrinsically its own end.

By always remaining a student with a "beginner's mind," the martial artist can eventually surpass himself because he learns to stand on the shoulders of his teachers, and profit from the cumulative wisdom and experiences of traditional martial arts masters. To maintain a sense of humility and a lifelong openness to learning is crucial no matter how long one has been training. The practitioner reminds himself: "Today I am better than I was yesterday, tomorrow I will be better still."

[The knight of faith] has drained the cup of life's
profound sadness, he knows the bliss of the infinite,
he senses the pain of renouncing everything,
the dearest things he possesses in the world,…
and yet he has this sense of security in enjoying it,
as though the finite life were the surest thing of all.
—Kierkegaard

To a free spirit, a free world.
—Taisen Deshimaru

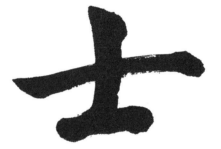

shih
knight

The Ultimate Convergence | XII

To become a true martial artist—to become a whole person—one goes through a long process of personal change and development. Change is not merely a series of points or events from the past to the present; in point of fact, it is a discontinuous trend. The Greeks had a metaphor of time in which the past is in front of us while the future sneaks up from behind us. What is intriguing about this reversal of a common perceptual experience of time is that it makes people think differently. When a person looks both ways in time, he discovers that he can only look forward as far as he can look back. The interweaving of the past-present-future pulls him along the thread of everyday life. The further along he moves along this continuum, the more he cherishes the conceit that the lessons learned from the past might yet inform and improve the world he leaves to his children. But the meaning of past events can be altered by what a person does today or what may happen in the future. Thus one is reminded of the interpretive circularities of the past-present-future. In this respect, if students and teachers can learn a new way to approach the martial arts, then they will have the ability and confidence to finally think and act for themselves. Martial arts instructors belong to a profession that is particularly susceptible to following the standard party line. The only cure for it is an injection of skepticism and independent thinking, an unwillingness to simply take things for granted.

A life of training and practice, a life pursued virtuously, is comprised of many, many days. But this kind of life can transform the banality and the petty servitude of the everyday into something intense, even dramatic. A personal world of empty space beckons to the brave soul who chooses to follow the path of the martial Way. This void demands to be filled with his knowledge and skills, hopes and fears, triumphs and disappointments, accomplishments and misadventures; and those of others in his life who gives his experience on this earth texture and meaning. His shared existence and the social interdependence with others are basic and constitutive. Only then can he emerge as a mature individual, having achieved a tiny portion of uniqueness, and stand tall with some nobility.

When an individual makes his journey through this constantly changing world, he leaves behind the baggage of convention and certainty, and enters a different, unfamiliar landscape. When he breaks from his life long daily routines and looks at the same things in a wholly different way, he has (as Don Juan described) stopped the world and started to see. The exhilaration of fulfilling his new potential is leavened by the attendant anxiety of walking into a realm of uncertainty. He is far from alone, because others have made this journey before, and more will do so in the future. But each person still has to find his own way through even if, at the end of it, he realizes that he has really traveled in a big circle and has merely come back home. Now he is finally at home with himself. He must not think that because his route was a circular one rather than a straight line, it meant that he was confused or inefficient. If there were a bright shining line that led directly to wisdom, he would not have been able to get on that path anyway because it would have been too crowded.

The martial Way is not linear but spherical. Its parts are related and each part has a bearing on the rest. There is no precise order to the practice of techniques, forms and other exercises. The life of the warrior is not merely theory and is not always comprehensible. Trying too hard to attain enlightenment is antithetical to the maintenance of a proper spirit, and thus a diffusion of effort and time. What the greatest philosophers can offer is not doctrine but dialectic, a conversation that impels each person in search of wisdom. This is a search in which men use their bodies, thoughts and senses to live and move with enlivened spirit and loftier purpose. There is no rest until we know what can be known, and why it is worth knowing.

When a man has completed this circle, he realizes that everything is done and there is nothing left to desire. There is no requirement to achieve some special state of mind, other than to realize his true nature. As Nietzsche said: "Become who you are." No profound introspection or mystical transcendence is required, just a clear-headed presence in the real world. All of the soul-searching and philosophizing, to paraphrase Wittgenstein, still "leaves the world as it is." It is profoundly surprising how relieved a man can be when he gives up the dogma of whatever spirituality or ideology that he has acquired to give himself a sense of structure and purpose. There is no system—theological, ideological or philosophical—that can make the world more certain or meaningful. Then he may realize that the truth lies in each individual's ordinary mind. When he has done this, he has everything, as if a veil covering an unseen world has just been lifted, revealing the mystery of life only to him. Likewise, when he loses it, he may also lose everything. His human nature may keep reminding him that there are still things he lacks which, if he could only possess them, would increase his strength, fame, wealth or happiness; but he intuitively knows that wanting more only creates restiveness, frustration and discontent. That if he tries to get it all, he only winds up striving for more. Desire engenders frustration, and frustrated desire brings on the enslavement of waiting for gratification.

How does a man let go of his own self-imposed reasoning? How does he know when he has enough? How does he transform the vicious circle into a virtuous circle? When the mind undergoes the process of self-discovery, it allows a man to go beyond the isolated boundaries of his own body. Yukio Mishima, Japan's most acclaimed novelist of the twentieth-century, was obsessed with living the samurai's *bushido* code, and with doing what was true to our nature. He viewed men's actions as "perishing with the blossom...[since] the imperishable flower is an artificial flower." So it may be impossible for an individual to completely abandon his self-centered desires, even as he tries his utmost to do so. However, by adhering to the martial Way, he can constantly refresh the insight that his money, his possessions and his physical self are only here to enjoy on a temporary basis. In time, they will all pass through his fingers and return from whence they came. The dualities of life that he wrestles with—profit and loss, victory and defeat, glory and shame—will all prove to be transient. Only such integrity can counterbalance the knowledge that a limited life is coming to a termination, and help a person face up to the despair and helplessness that marks the conscious end of an individual life.

Man is thrown into this world without his choice or knowledge. The world existed before he arrived and will likely remain unchanged after he departs. The ephemeral nature of his imperfect existence is never very far from his mind. But this very evanescence, like the momentary flash of light in the sky, is what gives his being its special character and strength. By brushing aside his pursuit of vanity and comfort, he also finds the means, with his last breath, to peacefully leave this material world behind. With sincerity and persistence, in a world defined by constant change, he can jettison false pride, self-conceit, and other weaknesses. Then he will know. Winning has nothing to do with arrogance and boastfulness. It has everything to do with a devotion to the path of understanding, for it is this path from which true content and grace will enter his life.

Martial arts practice helps the dedicated student to develop the strength and fortitude to face both life and death. The true martial artist knows that both happiness and tragedy must eventually come to an end. In *Hagakure*, he is reminded that human life lasts but an instant, just one brief shining moment in time. The martial artist as warrior is a myth that exists to inspire mere fallible mortals. It is an invitation for an individual to transform himself through practice and discipline. Philosophical reflection is an integral part of this way of life. He does not know if the end is tomorrow or many years from now. Yet he still must constantly think about what life might be like twenty years into the future. Time changes him, making him stronger or weaker as the case may be. He lives in a world of brute existence where not everything is possible; it is not a dream world. But if he lives each day aware that it might be his last, the ensuing twenty years will also pass like a dream. From moment to moment, from day to day, something will be accumulated that will enable him to better live in accordance with the philosophy of life that the martial Way teaches.

The martial artist does not seek to initiate aggression, but stands ready to use his skills to deter aggression. The real virtue of the martial Way is not to inflict harm upon another but, through practice and conditioning, to find an avenue through which he begins to know himself and from which life may open its secrets to him. The true warrior seeks to walk in peace while refraining from using his art. Along life's long journey, he is a solitary traveler who is neither moved by praise or criticism. He embodies the most worthy and dignified impulses of man and struggles to transcend the chaos and contradictions of the human condition. The warrior is not led by others; but by remaining true to his convictions, he may inspire others to follow in his steps. He chooses his path and gives us an example of the original and primary rule of life—how to learn, in order to be a man, to live and to die. Then he may gaze towards the sky, and in the immortal words of the English poet William Henley say to himself: "I am the master of my fate. I am the captain of my soul."

NOTES

I. The Force of Virtue

1. See Carlos Castaneda, *Journey To Ixtlan*, 1972. Castaneda's series of books on the lessons of an old Yaqui Indian named Don Juan Matos represent a classic literary vision of the world and a gateway to a profound way of thinking about oneself.
2. Castaneda, *Ibid.*, p. 107.
3. Popper, Karl. *The Open Society and its Enemies*, 1943. p. 200.

II. The Martial Way

4. The monumental tale *Three Kingdoms* offers a startling and unsparing view of how power is wielded, how diplomacy is conducted, and how wars are planned and fought. This Ming Dynasty masterpiece has influenced the way that Chinese think about power, diplomacy and war up to the current day.
5. Attributable to Francis Fukuyama's *The End of History and the Last Man*, (New York: Free Press, 1992), Chapter 28, "Men Without Chests."
6. From a famous excerpt in Nietzsche's *Twilight of the Idols* which was often quoted during his lifetime.
7. In *Karate-Do: My Way of Life*, See p. 77. Funakoshi describes his struggle to refine and popularize karate, and to sharpen the understanding of the art of self-defense and the means to personal longevity.
8. The *Phaedo* is the last testament of Socrates as told by Plato (*The Last Days of Socrates*, New York: Penguin, 1954).
9. Kierkegaard's *Concluding Unscientific Postscript* constitutes the turning point in his entire work as an author. It presents the problem of becoming a true Christian and is the starting point for the serious religious books that followed *Postscript*'s publication in 1848. This work stated in the clearest form yet the paradoxical implications of the Christian faith.
10. Casteneda, *Ibid.*, p. 54. With Don Juan as his informant, Casteneda recorded a student's initiation into the mysteries of sorcery, of becoming "a man of knowledge," of overcoming one's own fears, of "stopping the world" and "seeing" how one lives life.
11. Heidegger's *Being And Time*, originally published in 1927, is widely regarded as the most important Western philosophical work of the twentieth century. Its influence in philosophy, psychology and literature has literally changed the intellectual map of the modern world. In the translators J. Macquarrie and J. Robinson's preface to the first English edition of the work, they write: "It is safe to predict that now, more than ever, as life on earth becomes more precarious, Heidegger will become another way station in the restless pilgrimage of unhappy souls trying to find themselves."
12. In *Warrior Politics*, Robert Kaplan makes the historical and philosophical case that armed prophets such as Moses and Mohammed used self-interested ruthlessness and martial force to create and maintain moral and just institutions. He also incorporates the thinking of Aristotle, Sun-Tzu, Hobbes and Machiavelli to bolster his philosophical argument for the morality of lethal force.
13. Albert Camus' *The Rebel*, See p. 306., offers us a philosophy of politics in its examination of liberty and terror. It begins with a meditation on enduring or not enduring, on the implications of the act of resistance and rebellion. Published in 1956 with post-World War II Europe as its immediate backdrop, it is informed by a precise historical knowledge of the major developments of nineteenth and twentieth century Europe.

14. Kensho Furuya's *Kodo: Ancient Ways*, See p. 187., is a compilation of articles published between 1988 and 1995 in the magazine *Martial Arts Training*. His lessons are all inspired from the teachings of traditional martial arts and Buddhist sources. Furuya advocates embracing the martial arts traditions and practices as the means to true warrior training.

III. China Hand, Empty Hand

15. George Dillman, a 9th degree black belt in Ryukyu Kempo, was a National Karate Champion from 1969-1972. Dillman is best known for his system of pressure points and grappling that is embedded within traditional forms. As a result, he has opened up a formerly secret level of meaning in *kata* movements previously inaccessible to Western practitioners.

16. Based on research by Will Tracy who has done the most extensive original documentation of the historical origins and development of *kenpo karate*. See Will Tracy, *Tracy's Kenpo Karate*, 1998 (Unpublished).

17. The traditional system of *kenpo karate* has 533 techniques (including variations) and over 20 empty-hand and weapons forms. Traditional *kenpo* continues to be taught primarily by organizations and studios affiliated with Al and Will Tracy. Based in Louisville, Kentucky, the Tracy brothers were among the original *shodans* awarded by Ed Parker. The Tracy brothers eventually established their own network of member schools to promote the classical style of *kenpo* that they were trained in. In the years before Ed Parker's death in 1990, he created an abbreviated system of *kenpo* that became known as American *kenpo* to distinguish it from the much more extensive traditional system.

IV. No Magic Wand

18. Dave Lowry's *Moving Towards Stillness*, See p. 14., has been among the most articulate advocates of embracing the social values and moral imperatives of traditional martial arts, particularly the Japanese *budo* heritage. In his many works on training, he emphasizes the integration of martial arts principles into daily life.

VI. Lose Your Ego

19. Castaneda, *Ibid.* 1972.
20. Bruce Lee, *Tao of Jeet Kune Do*, 1975. p. 7.
21. Dave Lowry, *Moving Towards Stillness*, 2000.

VIII. The Illusion of Technique

22. Lee, *Ibid.*, p. 70.
23. The most difficult aspect of the advanced training of a martial artist is the development of spirit *(shen)* and energy *(chi)*. For a teacher to teach his student how to go "go beyond technique" requires the kind of discipleship that is described by Dang in his book *Beyond the Known*.

XI. Learning and Teaching

24. Casteneda, *Ibid.*
25. Furuya, *Ibid.*

BIBLIOGRAPHY

Camus, Albert. *The Rebel*. Translated by Justin O'Brien. Alfred A. Knopf: New York, NY, 1954.

Castaneda, Carlos. *A Separate Reality: Further Conversations with Don Juan*. Simon and Schuster: New York, NY, 1971.

Castaneda, Carlos. *Journey To Ixtlan: The Lessons of Don Juan*. Simon and Schuster: New York, NY, 1972.

Chuang Tzu. *The Complete Works of Chuang Tzu*. Columbia University Press: New York, NY, 1968.

Craig, Darrell Max. *Japan's Ultimate Martial Art*. Charles E. Tuttle Co.: Boston, MA, 1995.

Dang, Tri Thong. *Beyond the Known*. Charles E. Tuttle Co.: Boston, MA, 1993.

Deshimaru, Taisen. *The Zen Way To The Martial Arts*. Translated by Nancy Amphoux. E. P. Dutton Inc.: New York, NY, 1979.

Dillman, George with Chris Thomas. *Advanced Pressure Point Fighting of Ryuku Kempo*. George Dillman Karate International: Reading, PA, 1994.

Funakoshi, Gichin. *Karate-Do: My Way of Life*. Kodansha International: Tokyo, Japan, 1975.

Fukuyama, Francis. *The End of History and the Last Man*. Free Press: New York, NY, 1992.

Furuya, Kensho. *Kodo: Ancient Ways*. Ohara Publications: Santa Clarita, CA, 1996.

Hegel, G. W. F. *The Phenomenology of Mind*. Translated by J.B. Baillie. Harper: New York, 1967.

Heidegger, Martin. *Being And Time*. Translated by John Macquarrie and Edward Robinson. Harper & Row: New York, NY, 1962.

Herrigel, Eugen. *Zen In The Art of Archery*. Vintage Books: New York, NY, 1971.

Hoffman, Yoel (Translator). *The Sound of the One Hand: 281 Zen Koans with Answers*. Basic Book, Inc.: New York, NY, 1975.

Hyams, Joe. *Zen In The Martial Arts*. G.P. Putnam: New York, NY, 1979.

Jou, Tsung Hwa. *The Tao of I Ching*. Tai Chi Foundation. Distributed by Charles E. Tuttle Co.: Boston, MA, 1984.

Kaplan, Robert D. *Warrior Politics: Why Leadership Demands a Pagan Ethos*. Random House: New York, NY: 2001.

Kaufman, Stephen F. *The Living Tao: Meditations on the Tao Te Ching to Empower Your Life*. Charles E. Tuttle Co.: Boston, MA, 1998.

Kierkegaard, Soren. *Concluding Unscientific Postscript*. Translated by David F. Swenson and Walter Lowrie. Princeton University Press: Princeton, NJ, 1941.

Kierkegaard, Soren. *Fear and Trembling*. Translated by Walter Lowrie. Princeton University Press: Princeton, NJ, 1941.

Lao Tzu. *Tao Te Ching*. Penguin Books: New York, NY, 1963.

Lee, Bruce. *Tao of Jeet Kune Do*. Ohara Publications: Santa Clarita, CA, 1975.

Lowry, Dave. *Moving Toward Stillness*. Tuttle Publishing: Boston, MA, 2000.

Luo, Guanzhong. *Three Kingdoms*. Translated by Moss Roberts. Foreign Language Press/University of California Press: Beijing, People's Republic of China, 1994.

Mishima, Yukio. *Hagakure Nyumon (The Way of the Samurai)*. Translated by Kathryn Sparling. Basic Books: New York, NY, 1977.

Mitose, James M. *What Is Self Defense? (Kenpo Jiu-Jitsu)*. Kosho-Shorei Publishing Co.: Sacramento, CA, 1953.

Musashi, Miyamoto. *A Book Of Five Rings: A Guide to Strategy*. Translated by Victor Harris. The Overlook Press: Woodstock, NY, 1974.

Nietzsche, Friedrich. *The Will to Power*. Translated by Walter Kaufmann and R. J. Hollingdale. Vintage Books: New York, NY, 1968.

Parker, Ed. *Kenpo Karate: Law Of The Fist And The Empty Hand*. Delsby Publications: Los Angeles, CA, 1960.

Plato. *The Last Days of Socrates*. Translated by Hugh Tredennick. Penguin: New York, 1954.

Popper, Karl R. *The Open Society and its Enemies, Volume I*. Princeton University Press: Princeton, NJ, 1943.

Sun Tzu. *The Art of War*. Translated by Lionel Giles. Guo Huang Publishing Co., Taipei, Taiwan, R.O.C.: 1985.

Suzuki, Shunryu. *Zen Mind, Beginner's Mind*. John Weatherhill, Inc.: New York, NY, 1970.

Tohei, Koichi. *Ki In Daily Life*. Ki No Kenkyukai H.Q.: Tokyo, Japan, 1978.

Tracy, Will. *Tracy's Kenpo Karate*. Unpublished, 1998.

Ueshiba, Morihei. *Budo: Teachings of the Founder of Aikido*. Translated by John Stevens. Kodansha International: Tokyo, Japan, 1991.

Waley, Arthur. *The Analects of Confucius*. Translated and annotated by Arthur Waley. George Allen & Unwin Ltd.: London, U.K., 1938.

Waley, Arthur. *Three Ways of Thought In Ancient China*. Macmillan Co.: New York, NY, 1939.

Wu, Wai Hong. *The Heritage of Fu-Jow Pai (Tiger Claw)*. The Fu-Jow Pai Federation, Inc.: New York, NY, 1979.

Yamamoto, Tsunetomo. *Hagakure: The Book of the Samurai*. Translated by William Scott Nelson. Kodansha International: Tokyo, Japan, 1979.

INDEX

ABOUT THE AUTHOR

F. J. Chu, born in Taiwan, Republic of China, is a certified black belt instructor in kenpo karate and has trained in other martial arts styles including fu jow pai (tiger claw kung fu) and aikido over the last twenty-five years.

Chu is President of Sage Capital Group, Inc. (an investment management firm), and has held directorships in numerous public and private companies and industry organizations. He is also the Principal of the Chinese School of Southern Westchester in Scarsdale, New York. Chu is a graduate of Yale College, where he studied philosophy and psychology, and the Harvard Business School.

An author of two previous books *Paradigm Lost: The Psychology of Money and Investing* (2001), *The Mind of the Market* (1999), Chu has published many articles in professional and academic journals.

Chu lives with his wife and three children in Rye, New York. In addition to his martial arts, writing and business activities, he is a Councilman on the Rye City Council and a 2003 graduate of the Westchester County Citizens Police Academy. He serves on the Board of Directors of the United Way of Westchester and Putnam, the Mental Health Association of Westchester County and the Organization of Chinese Americans.

朱嘉年者

COMPLETE BOOKS FROM YMAA

COMPLETE VIDEOTAPES FROM YMAA

more products available from...
YMAA Publication Center, Inc. 楊氏東方文化出版中心
4354 Washington Street Roslindale, MA 02131
1-800-669-8892 • ymaa@aol.com • www.ymaa.com

COMPLETE VIDEOTAPES FROM YMAA (CONTINUED)

CHIN NA IN DEPTH—COURSE 4	T039/035
CHIN NA IN DEPTH—COURSE 5	T040/124
CHIN NA IN DEPTH—COURSE 6	T041/132
CHIN NA IN DEPTH—COURSE 7	T044/965
CHIN NA IN DEPTH—COURSE 8	T045/973
CHIN NA IN DEPTH—COURSE 9	T047/548
CHIN NA IN DEPTH—COURSE 10	T048/556
CHIN NA IN DEPTH—COURSE 11	T051/564
CHIN NA IN DEPTH—COURSE 12	T052/572
CHINESE QIGONG MASSAGE—SELF	T008/327
CHINESE QIGONG MASSAGE—PARTNER	T009/335
COMP. APPLICATIONS OF SHAOLIN CHIN NA 1	T012/386
COMP. APPLICATIONS OF SHAOLIN CHIN NA 2	T013/394
DEFEND YOURSELF 1—UNARMED	T010/343
DEFEND YOURSELF 2—KNIFE	T011/351
EMEI BAGUAZHANG 1	T017/280
EMEI BAGUAZHANG 2	T018/299
EMEI BAGUAZHANG 3	T019/302
EIGHT SIMPLE QIGONG EXERCISES FOR HEALTH 2ND ED.	T005/54X
ESSENCE OF TAIJI QIGONG	T006/238
MUGAI RYU	T050/467
NORTHERN SHAOLIN SWORD—SAN CAI JIAN & ITS APPLICATIONS	T035/051
NORTHERN SHAOLIN SWORD—KUN WU JIAN & ITS APPLICATIONS	T036/06X
NORTHERN SHAOLIN SWORD—QI MEN JIAN & ITS APPLICATIONS	T037/078
QIGONG: 15 MINUTES TO HEALTH	T042/140
SCIENTIFIC FOUNDATION OF CHINESE QIGONG—LECTURE	T029/590
SHAOLIN KUNG FU BASIC TRAINING - 1	T057/0045
SHAOLIN KUNG FU BASIC TRAINING - 2	T058/0053
SHAOLIN LONG FIST KUNG FU—LIEN BU CHUAN	T002/19X
SHAOLIN LONG FIST KUNG FU—GUNG LI CHUAN	T003/203
SHAOLIN LONG FIST KUNG FU—ER LU MAI FU	T014/256
SHAOLIN LONG FIST KUNG FU—SHI ZI TANG	T015/264
SHAOLIN LONG FIST KUNG FU—TWELVE TAN TUI	T043/159
SHAOLIN LONG FIST KUNG FU—XIAO HU YAN	T025/604
SHAOLIN WHITE CRANE GONG FU—BASIC TRAINING 1	T046/440
SHAOLIN WHITE CRANE GONG FU—BASIC TRAINING 2	T049/459
SIMPLIFIED TAI CHI CHUAN—24 & 48	T021/329
SUN STYLE TAIJIQUAN	T022/469
TAI CHI CHUAN & APPLICATIONS—24 & 48	T024/485
TAIJI BALL QIGONG - 1	T054/475
TAIJI BALL QIGONG - 2	T057/483
TAIJI BALL QIGONG - 3	T062/0096
TAIJI BALL QIGONG - 4 MARTIAL APPLICATIONS	T063/010X
TAIJI CHIN NA	T016/408
TAIJI PUSHING HANDS - 1	T055/505
TAIJI PUSHING HANDS - 2	T058/513
TAIJI PUSHING HANDS - 3	T064/0134
TAIJI PUSHING HANDS - 4	T065/0142
TAIJI PUSHING HANDS - 5	T066/0150
TAIJI SABER	T053/491
TAIJI & SHAOLIN STAFF - FUNDAMENTAL TRAINING - 1	T061/0088
TAIJI SWORD, CLASSICAL YANG STYLE	T031/817
TAIJI YIN & YANG SYMBOL STICKING HANDS–YANG TAIJI TRAINING	T056/580
TAIJI YIN & YANG SYMBOL STICKING HANDS–YIN TAIJI TRAINING	T067/0177
TAIJIQUAN, CLASSICAL YANG STYLE	T030/752
WHITE CRANE HARD QIGONG	T026/612
WHITE CRANE SOFT QIGONG	T027/620
WILD GOOSE QIGONG	T032/949
WU STYLE TAIJIQUAN	T023/477
XINGYIQUAN—12 ANIMAL FORM	T020/310
YANG STYLE TAI CHI CHUAN	T001/181

COMPLETE DVDS FROM YMAA

ANALYSIS OF SHAOLIN CHIN NA (DVD)	DVD012/0231
CHIN NA INDEPTH COURSES 1 - 4 (DVD)	DVD001/602
CHIN NA INDEPTH COURSES 5 - 8 (DVD)	DVD004/610
CHIN NA INDEPTH COURSES 9 - 12 (DVD)	DVD005/629
EIGHT SIMPLE QIGONG EXERCISES FOR HEALTH (DVD)	DVD008/0037
ESSENCE OF TAIJI QIGONG (DVD)	DVD010/0215
SHAOLIN KUNG FU FUNDAMENTAL TRAINING - 1&2 (DVD)	DVD009/0207
SHAOLIN LONG FIST KUNG FU - BASIC SEQUENCES (DVD)	DVD007/661
SHAOLIN WHITE CRANE GONG FU BASIC TRAINING 1 & 2	DVD006/599
TAIJIQUAN CLASSICAL YANG STYLE (DVD)	DVD002/645
TAIJI SWORD, CLASSICAL YANG STYLE (DVD)	DVD011/0223
WHITE CRANE HARD & SOFT QIGONG (DVD)	DVD003/637

more products available from...

YMAA Publication Center, Inc. 楊氏東方文化出版中心

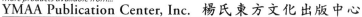

4354 Washington Street Roslindale, MA 02131
1-800-669-8892 • ymaa@aol.com • www.ymaa.com